The World According to Kemosabe

Tigger Montague

Copyright © 2017 Tigger Montague

ISBN: 978-1-63492-838-0

All rights reserved. No part of this publication may be reproduced, stored in a retrieval system, or transmitted in any form or by any means, electronic, mechanical, recording or otherwise, without the prior written permission of the author.

Published by BookLocker.com, Inc., St. Petersburg, Florida.

Printed on acid-free paper.

The characters and events in this book are fictitious. Any similarity to real persons, living or dead, is coincidental and not intended by the author.

BookLocker.com, Inc.
2017

First Edition

DISCLAIMER

This book details the author's personal experiences with and opinions about canine nutrition. The author is not a healthcare provider.

The author and publisher are providing this book and its contents on an "as is" basis and make no representations or warranties of any kind with respect to this book or its contents. The author and publisher disclaim all such representations and warranties, including for example warranties of merchantability and healthcare for a particular purpose. In addition, the author and publisher do not represent or warrant that the information accessible via this book is accurate, complete or current.

The statements made about products and services have not been evaluated by the U.S. Food and Drug Administration. They are not intended to diagnose, treat, cure, or prevent any condition or disease. Please consult with your own physician or healthcare specialist regarding the suggestions and recommendations made in this book.

Except as specifically stated in this book, neither the author or publisher, nor any authors, contributors, or other representatives will be liable for damages arising out of or in connection with the use of this book. This is a comprehensive limitation of liability that applies to all damages of any kind, including (without limitation) compensatory; direct, indirect or consequential damages; loss of data, income or profit; loss of or damage to property and claims of third parties.

You understand that this book is not intended as a substitute for consultation with a licensed healthcare practitioner, such as your physician. Before you begin any healthcare program, or change your lifestyle in any way, you will consult your physician or other licensed healthcare practitioner to ensure that you are in good health and that the examples contained in this book will not harm you.

This book provides content related to topics physical and/or mental health issues. As such, use of this book implies your acceptance of this disclaimer.

This book is dedicated to my mom, Cinnie, whose never-ending support and unconditional love allowed me to blaze my own trail.

Kemosabe dedicates this book to his mom, Soundtrack's Custom D'Zine, whose love he carries with him always.

In Memoriam

The Dogs of My Lifetime

Schylur
Spike
Nikki
Mei Mei
Kojak
Bear Dog
Skye Dog
Wookie the Wonder Dog
Kizzie
Toby
Hawkeye
Ravenwolf
Sierra
Rocky Raccoon
Jar Jar Binks
Rutrow
Spirit Dog

Table of Contents

Preface XI

Introduction 1

Part I: The Storyteller's Tales 5

    T-Bone and the Fence Testers 7
    Wolves at the Door 12
    The Power of the Bark Side 23
    Spirit Dog 39
    Fowl Play 53
    I Herd You 65
    The Reverend Mr. Schmoo 80

Part II: Nutrition and Recipes 87

    Food, Glorious Food 89
    Chow Time: What Do I Feed My Dog? 101
    How We Got to Kibble 117
    Dog Food Allergies 127
    Feeding the Overweight Dog 133
    Feeding for Healthy Skin and Coat 139
    Bone Broth 149
    Feeding for the Kidneys 151
    Feeding for the Liver 157
    Feeding for the Pancreas 163
    Feeding the Diabetic Dog 169
    Feeding Dogs with Cancer 173
    Feeding Puppies 187

    Going Raw 197
    Seeking the Balance 207
    Warming, Cooling, and Neutral Foods 211
    Bovine Colostrum for Canines 215
    Supplements 219

Part III: Kemosabe's Point of View 223

    Mealtime 225
    Bison for Breakfast 229
    Lassi (not Lassie) 231
    Aliens Among Us 235
    Living with Cats 239
    On the Road Again 243
    Rescue Me 249
    Skunked 253
    The Puppy Cometh 257
    When Bad Stress Happens to Good Dogs 261
    Canine Tips for Happy Holidays 265
    Food for the Holidays 269

Appendix A: Home-Cooked Recipes 273

Appendix B: More Tips on Feeding Raw 279

Appendix C: Product Recommendations 287

Acknowledgements 297

Bibliography 299

About the Author 305

Index 307

Preface

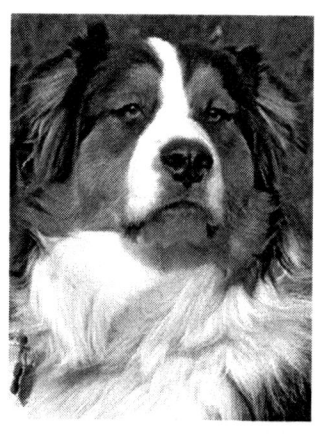

My name is Kemosabe. I am also known as 'Sabe, 'Sabe-Come, 'Sabe-Leave-It, and Monkey Boy. I am the Storyteller of the Springdale Tribe. Being a storyteller is an important role in every tribe, pack, and family. A storyteller is an historian, observer, a verbal documentarian, and commentator. In the canine world, a storyteller keeps not only the stories of the dogs, but of the humans and other animals in our environment. It's a big job—one that has been handed down from our earliest beginnings as wolves. Humans don't realize this, but a lone howling wolf is often a storyteller, singing the tales to the moon and the pack.

My tribe is made up of a canine breed called the Australian shepherd, also known simply as Aussies. Despite our name we did not originate from Australia. We are an American breed, developed in the 1800s to herd Australian sheep imported into the western states of the US. We are known for our intelligence, which includes outsmarting our humans, and for our work ethic and stamina. Australian shepherds excel at herding, agility, flyball, frisbee, and obedience. We can work as therapy dogs, in search and rescue, and as assistance dogs. Most importantly we are loyal and loving and appreciate a nice soft couch or comfy overstuffed chair: with or without the human.

It is important for an Australian shepherd to have a job. If the human doesn't create a job for us, we will create one for ourselves or become bored and destructive. Sometimes Aussies end up in shelters or rescues because their human didn't understand that we are working dogs, we need to work.

My tribe consists of five canines: Cake Walk, Thunderbear, Buckaroo, Crockett, and me. Cake Walk is the only girl of the pack, but we don't treat her any differently until she gets tired of playing Boy Games with us and then, just like our mothers, she gets in our face and tells us off. If you live with a human female you know what I mean.

We live on a farm in Virginia that includes horses and chickens and two alien beings known as cats. There are deer, fox, possums, raccoons, squirrels, wild turkeys, the occasional black bear, and a roving band of coyotes. There are creeks, a small pond, forest and fields, so we have plenty of space to run and swim and chase wild critters.

We live with two humans. One human is a female and we call her Boss Lady, although she functions as our housekeeper, attendant, groomer, nurse, chauffeur, dietician, and wait staff. The other human is male and we call him Peter. He functions as our butler, valet, chef, home repairman, and resident philosopher.

Boss Lady has a company called BioStar, which makes whole food supplements for horses and dogs. This is very advantageous for the Aussie Tribe because we get to taste-test every product. We also get to go to work with Boss Lady, hang around the production area where the products are made, and sweep the floor clean of any remnants. I have been known to steal the BioStar cookie bars as they are being taken out of the dehydrators.

Peter is retired and runs the farm. He always carries treats in his pockets, which makes him very popular with the Tribe. Cake Walk is Peter's dog and she never fails to remind us of that fact.

This book is the collection of a storyteller's tales as well as the information from Boss Lady about food and nutrition for dogs, how to support specific canine health challenges with foods and plants, and some of my personal observations on life with humans, cats, and horses.

Some of the stories are those that were passed down to me from Spirit Dog, the Tribe's previous storyteller. Spirit Dog learned the stories from Rocky Raccoon, Jar-Jar Binks, and Ravenwolf, who learned from Bear Dog, Kojak, Mei Mei, and Nikki. These stories aren't just our stories; they are our humans' stories too.

Introduction

by Tigger Montague

Canine nutrition can be a rather dry subject. There are many, many good books on canine nutrition, and I doubted I could write about the subject any better than previous authors.

For the last thirty years I have lived on a farm with multiple dogs—a venerable pack, a motley crew of canine personalities. Some dogs were rescues, some adopted from the SPCA, some purchased as puppies from breeders. Some were challenging, some were entertaining, some owned me lock, stock, and barrel. Every single one of them was a teacher with paws.

Many years ago, while watching the dogs lying close to one another under the shade of the walnut trees, all of them awake but relaxed, it occurred to me how much like a human tribe they were: there was a leader, there were warriors, and there was the storyteller, the one who remembers, who re-tells and passes on the stories of the tribe. Every pack member, new and old, lay under those walnut trees hearing the stories and adventures of pack members long gone, as well as current tales of hunts, humans, chickens, and cats.

In writing this book on nutrition, I wanted to include my canine tribe's stories—and who better to tell those stories than their current Storyteller, Kemosabe? Together we collaborated on the book, with me handling the nutrition section, and he sharing the stories of the pack as well as his own personal viewpoints on things.

The book is divided into four sections: The Storyteller's Tales, Nutrition and Recipes, Kemosabe's Point of View, and a set of appendices that includes helpful tips, guidelines, and recommendations for feeding a raw diet, along with recipes for home-cooked meals for dogs.

Over a lifetime shared with dogs, there are the very special ones, the dogs who become our best friends. The dogs we love deeply and profoundly. Their hearts speaks to our hearts, and we are forever changed by it. Kemosabe is one of those dogs.

I hope there is a Kemosabe in your life, or a new puppy that will become your storyteller, the dog of your heart.

The World According to Kemosabe

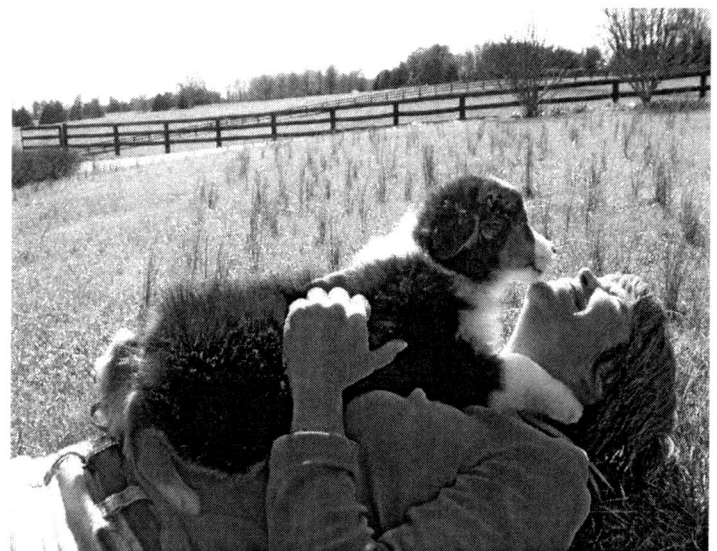

Tigger and The Storyteller as a puppy

Part I

The Storyteller's Tales

T-Bone and the Fence Testers

This story was told to me by Rocky Raccoon, who heard it from Wookie, who heard it from Skye Dog. It is one of the Tribe's favorite stories because we think it is one of the reasons Boss Lady got into herding dogs.

Before my time, Boss Lady was married to Angry Man. When they moved to Virginia, they bought a farm, and part of the purchase included: one black pony named Pootie, one steer, three cows, and a heifer.

Angry man didn't know anything about farming. He was a city boy. Boss Lady had spent her youth running around her grandparents farm, playing with lambs, and riding ponies at a small boarding and lesson barn. She was so horse-crazy she would do anything to ride...and did once decide, with a childhood friend, to ride a very large bovine in the neighbor's field. The girls named their new friend Ringnose because of the obvious ring in the nose. They would get on their bikes to meet up at Mr. Fisher's farm, and give Ringnose treats like carrots and apples. When they had figured the bovine was pretty tame, they brought a halter and lead rope, climbed on from the fence and took turns riding Ringnose around the pasture.

One day Boss Lady came home and told her mother she had ridden a nice cow in Mr. Fisher's field and that she and her friend had named the cow Ringnose. Her mother, not normally prone to swooning, let out a shriek equal to that of any in a Hollywood horror film.

"That is not a cow, that is a *bull*!"

"Ringnose is nice, Mom. He wouldn't hurt me."

"Don't let me ever catch you riding that animal again or you will be very, very sorry."

So for bovine experience, Boss Lady had Ringnose and that was about it. Still, it was a lot more experience than Angry Man had. One early, frosty Saturday morning two months after Boss Lady and Angry Man moved to the farm, Boss Lady looked outside to see the steer, cows and heifer in the front yard. Angry Man was passed out asleep from the copious amounts of alcohol he had consumed the night before. She knew that waking him would mean certain consequences including rage and recriminations.

She threw a jacket over her pajamas, slipped on her boots, and went outside. The bovines were unperturbed by her presence. Huge cow patties had sprouted up all over the lawn. She walked out to the barn with the two dogs, Bear and Skye, who were young mixed breeds from the SPCA and had no herding genes. She grabbed a bucket, threw some grain in it, and walked back to the lawn shaking the bucket.

The bovines looked at her. She shook the bucket again. One of the cows responded by taking a bite out of a late blooming rose. The steer started to walk towards her, which caused Bear and Skye to bark, which spooked the bovines and caused them to head down the driveway, not quite at a stampede pace.

Horsewomen are, by necessity, resourceful. The bovines had stopped moving because they found some patches of grass along the fence lines of the driveway. Boss Lady circled around them by going through one of the pastures so that she could get in front of the animals, open the gate on the left side of the drive and let them back into the field. As she slipped through the fence boards she felt resistance and heard the lovely sound of fabric ripping. She shook the bucket again and then starting leaving a breadcrumb trail of grain for the Hansel and Gretel bovines to follow. The steer caught on. As soon as he starting following the grain bits, the cows and heifer followed too, and eventually they were all back in the field.

Of course, getting the bovines back in the pasture was one thing. Figuring out where they had escaped was another. With Bear and Skye, she started to walk the fence lines, and then she saw it: two posts and three boards down...a huge section of fence, demolished. The bovines, knowing that the grass is greener on the other side, began moving again towards their new escape hatch.

There are a lot of things to be said about Boss Lady, but being deft with hammer and nails is not one of them. She considered stringing some lunge lines across the opening, then briefly thought about duct taping the broken posts to the rotted post still left in the ground, and then wondered if calling 911 or the fire department would be helpful. She ended up doing what every other horsewoman would do:

she got in the big Ford Dually and parked it in front of the broken fence.

Boss Lady climbed out of the truck to make sure the heifer couldn't sneak through some gap, and stood there in that cold morning air, her flannel pajama bottoms wet from the grass, her feet cold from putting on boots without socks, the unmistakable odor of cow dung on the soles, hair unbrushed with bits of feed in it from the bovine roundup, and her barn jacket oozing its synthetic lining from several small tears in the fabric.

Bear and Skye started barking. She looked around and then heard the sound...a vehicle approaching at 7:30 in the morning. Her neighbor, the retired Sergeant Major of the Marine Corps, was coming up the drive. The Sergeant Major lived in a house that sat on a hill with views of the long farm driveway.

To her credit, she didn't run like a banshee into the house, nor did she slink silently into the barn to hide in a stall. She leaned against the truck as if she always leaned against the truck in the mornings, because that's what horsewomen do, and waved to her neighbor as he called out.

"Morning! Saw your cows got out, wondered if you needed any help."

"I got them back in," Boss Lady said.

He got out of his car, took a good look at the truck and how it was parallel parked, and said, "I've got some posts and fence boards. How 'bout we fix this fence?" He walked over to the fence line and looked at the bovines. "You could get some mighty fine T-bone steaks out of that steer."

Boss Lady cocked her head and smiled. The bovines became known as T-Bone and the Fence Testers from then on. That steer ended up being not quite a steer, but a bull with one testicle, as evidenced by the two cows that gave birth the following spring.

Boss Lady ended up a vegetarian.

Wolves at the Door

Part Malamute, part Canadian timber wolf, he weighed 140 pounds—a massive creature who, despite his size, moved with cat-like softness. He was behind you before you realized it. He could stand next to a car and look at the driver through the window. It was a habit found unsettling by the mailman who, more than once, threw the mail on the ground and roared out of the driveway.

She was white and a mere 70 pounds, part wolf, part German shepherd. She was clever, sneaky even, always able to figure things out. She loved to sing: to the humans, to the sky, to the wildness within her. She would tilt her head back and release a mezzo-soprano voice, at times tinged with joy, and other times a deep longing. When she sang, the rest of the pack would join in. Of course some of the pack members weren't really singers; they were barkers and yippers doing their best to accompany her.

Boss Lady referred these to the canine/wolf choruses as Sing Fests, and she would join in, howling in an alto voice and a slightly different key.

His name was Ravenwolf, and hers was Sierra. They were known as Raven and Sweetie. Raven had come as a four-month-old pup to the farm, but Sierra was over a year old when she came to live in the pack. She had been living with two University of Virginia students who kept her in a first floor apartment. She hated confinement; she kept ripping out the window screens and jumping out. At the farm, she had freedom and a group of dogs she could lead. She also figured out how to open screen doors to let herself out, and never jumped out of another window.

As a puppy, Raven figured out potty training within a week, but due to his voracious appetite managed to consume half a leather couch, part of the footboard of Boss Lady's four-poster bed, a pleather jacket, a leather halter, two cushions, several books, and one leg of a dining room chair. Boss Lady often referred to him as the Beaver.

As he outgrew puppyhood, he emerged into a very large dog. School bus-size, the humans said. He took up so much space in the house, the pack thought of him as a kind of whale-wolf-dog. He made the average Malamute look like a small Eskimo Spitz in comparison. He intimidated not only the mailman, but the UPS and FedEx drivers too, as he just stood there, blocking the driver's side door, a huge immovable creature. Fact is, he was looking for treats. Wasn't that, after all, the reason that humans existed?

One day a strange car drove slowly up the farm drive. Boss Lady was in the kitchen at the sink, and looked out the window to see a sheriff's car pull over on the grass near the back door. Raven had ambled over to the car and stood looking at the driver. The other dogs milled around barking.

The driver honked his horn. Always slightly suspicious of law enforcement from her days as a hippie, she stayed at the sink looking out the window. The car's electric window opened slowly, and a flurry of small brown things were ejected out the window towards the dogs, who dispersed from their congregation around the car, chasing after the flying objects. Boss Lady ran out of the kitchen and out to the sheriff's car, a part of her mind running through a checklist of laws she had probably broken in the last 60 days including speeding, tailgating, passing from the right lane, and purchasing half an ounce of cannabis for a party.

The deputy smiled sheepishly. What he had been throwing were dog treats.

"I've heard about this farm and your dogs," he said. "I came prepared."

He handed her a subpoena to testify in a court case involving a motor vehicle accident she had witnessed. The sigh of relief from Boss Lady could be felt by every canine in the pack. Raven sniffed the envelope to make sure no treats were hidden inside.

"You've got a good alarm system here, with all these dogs," the deputy said.

"I know," she smiled.

"Well, have a nice day," he said, and rolled up his window and headed down the drive. Raven followed the car until it passed the old hay barn, as was his custom, to ensure the stranger was leaving. He watched as the car headed down the hill. Humans were so unpredictable. And who knows, there could be more flying treats.

***

Raven and Sweetie patrolled a territory larger than the farm itself. Some of the pack members said it went north to the little bridge over the wide part of the creek, and others said it included all of the hundreds of acres owned by the West Virginia Paper Company to the south and west of the farm. However large it was, the wolf-dogs spent time managing their territory. They liked to work after breakfast, and then again at night, after dinner, heading off to ensure the boundaries were maintained, that foxes and raccoons were properly treed, and deer were chased out of the glades for the sheer joy of the run.

There were trophies. Raven dragged back half a deer carcass, a couple of legs, and a head on separate excursions. The other pack members thought it was an amazing act of largesse, this sharing of the bounty of venison. Boss Lady did not share this viewpoint, and was quick with a shovel and rocks to bury the remains.

She often wondered where exactly her wolf-dogs went on their excursions. She could see them trotting off towards the neighbor houses on the south side of the farm property, see them slip through the fences, or in Raven's case clear them with a running leap. Neighborhood dogs would bark, but the wolf-dogs took no notice. They just kept moving until they were out of sight.

On a cold December afternoon, three days before Christmas, and the day before Boss Lady was to fly out to visit family in Arizona, a three-year-old warmblood filly named Nimahway busted through a pasture fence, followed by several other horses and an ancient forty-year-old Chincoteague pony known as Grandma, whose sight and hearing were fading away. Nimahway headed down the driveway with the others following and then veered through the open gate of a neighbor's pasture. Boss Lady got a bucket of feed, put a halter on one of the adult horses, and led them back to one of the smaller paddocks. Raven followed her with Sweetie behind him. As Boss Lady led the horses into the paddock, Nimahway bolted away and ran back down the driveway with Grandma right behind her. The filly and pony got to the road, turned right, and galloped up to the dirt road where the neighboring farm was.

Boss Lady grabbed her bucket, a halter, and headed for the dirt road with Raven by her side. It was cold, and the wind had picked up. The pony and filly kept trotting down the road, and due to the thick forest on either side there was no way to get around the duo and turn them around. Following only increased their forward movement.

Finally, a mile or so down the road, Grandma spied something to eat on the lawn of a small cabin. It had now turned dark, and lights glowed from inside the cabin, along with the sound of laughter...maybe a party?

The food bucket enticed Nimahway to come, the halter was slipped on, and Boss Lady draped the belt from her jeans around Grandma's neck. They began the walk home with Raven in the lead, taking his long, soft steps, familiar territory as this was to him. He knew the old dirt road like the back of his paw.

Boss Lady led Nimahway and Grandma down the farm neighbor's drive and to the gate. Mission Accomplished, she thought to herself, feeling the adrenalin begin to dissipate now that she was so close to home and the crisis was over. She fumbled with the gate chain in her cold hands as she held on to the pony and the mare. Realizing she needed one free set of fingers, she let go of Grandma. In that second the pony bolted away and trotted off towards the dirt road as the belt around her neck slipped to the ground. Nimahway leaped, but Boss Lady held on, the mare then screamed for Grandma, bucked, and threw her head in the equine version of a two-year-old child's meltdown.

Boss Lady hung on to the lead rope and the hysterical Nimahway, weighing her options in nano seconds: go after Grandma with Nimahway in tow, or put Nimahway back in the pasture with the others and go get Grandma. She decided to take care of Nimahway first. As she led the frantic Nimahway towards the paddock she looked behind to see Raven trotting away in pursuit of Grandma.

With the young mare still screaming for Grandma in the paddock, Boss Lady got in her car, drove to the dirt road, and saw in her headlights the pony, followed by Raven. She pulled over and started on foot, leaving the car running for the headlight illumination. It was a pitch-black by now. She had a 6:00 a.m. flight out, and had not yet packed for her trip. She had not yet written the feeding instructions for the barn sitter, the dogs and cats had not been fed, there was laundry to do, dishes to wash, last-minute gifts to wrap, she really needed to pee, and she had forgotten to bring the feed bucket this time.

She stopped walking and looked up at the sky, the winter stars blinking in the cold air. She had wanted the divorce, she had wanted freedom from the angry man she had married. But now, on the side of the road, following a half-blind pony and a wolf-dog in the dark and cold, being alone didn't feel like freedom. It felt like an enormous burden.

She reached the slope in the road, and there was no more illumination from the car. Only the stars gave light. Her eyes adjusted to the dark, to the tree shapes on the side of the road, and she saw house lights ahead, smiling at her, beckoning warmth. Her hands were cold, her feet were cold, and some internal power source kept her moving towards the dark shapes on the road: Grandma and Raven.

She heard the car before she saw the lights. It was moving fast, as cars do when the driver sees only an empty country road. Boss Lady's heart thumped like a jackhammer. Would the car see Grandma? Would it slow down? Stop? Hit her?

Raven moved to the middle of the road and stood there like a statue. The breaks squealed, the horn sounded, and Boss Lady waved her arms and yelled: "Please stop!"

The car swerved and came to a stop. Grandma was still walking, unperturbed. Boss Lady and Raven approached the vehicle. Raven walked up and looked at the 17-year-old driver through the window.

"That's a big dog," the boy said.

"Could you do me a favor?" Boss Lady asked. "Back your car up and park it so that it blocks the road and I can catch the pony."

"What pony?" The driver didn't take his eyes off Raven.

"There's a small pony walking on the edge of the road. I need to catch her."

The car flew into reverse and started backing up as Raven and Boss Lady followed. She saw Grandma seconds before the driver saw her too, and swung the car around to block Grandma's forward progress. The pony stopped within inches of the car's rear fender. Raven trotted up and made himself a wall between the pony and the woods.

Boss Lady swung the lead rope over the pony's neck and thanked the driver, who then drove away slowly, convinced that a night starting out like this one was bound to get even weirder.

Raven trotted ahead as they walked back down the road, stopped while Boss Lady turned her car off and grabbed the keys, then continued on to the neighbor's farm, through the gates, and back to the paddocks. There was still a broken fence to fix before she could turn the horses out in the big pasture, there was more hay to put out, and her car was still on the dirt road. She knew the fence boards were toast, so she parked the pickup truck to block the broken section, turned the horses out, put out more hay, tucked Nimahway and Grandma into their stalls, and set out with Raven to get the car.

As soon as she had turned on the ignition and the headlights, she saw Raven: heading down the road once again, then slipping into a driveway. She thought she heard him woof, but chalked it up to exhaustion and turned the car around to go home. Little did she know that a woman in the house at the end of that driveway opened her door and greeted the wolf-dog with, "Big Boy, you almost missed your treat," patted the big head and gave him the patty from a MacDonald's hamburger.

* * *

Many years later when Raven passed away, one of the neighbors, the Sergeant Major, drove up and asked Boss Lady where the "big dog" was. She told him of Raven's passing.

"He had quite a racket goin' on," the Sergeant Major said. "He and the white one would make the rounds, get food, and move on to the next house. I hear they'd go all the way down to Mrs. Baxter's place, you know, where the road dead-ends. She said they liked her ham and pea soup."

Boss Lady smiled and wiped her eyes. Sweetie walked up slowly and looked at the man as he continued.

"That big dog—I got my gun out the first time I saw him walkin' my fence line, but the wife, she said he's not botherin' nothin', let him be. I was afraid he might kill that little dog of Mrs. Roberts', but the big dog totally ignored that little poodle. Now the white one there," he said, pointing to Sweetie, "the white one, she's sneaky. Pulled chicken off my grill one day when I went into the house to get more barbecue sauce."

"Yes, she is a very clever," Boss Lady nodded.

"I worried about Big Dog," the man said. "Him and White One running free like that, even with collars and tags."

"They're part wolf," Boss Lady said. "There's something innately wild in them...not wild as in dangerous, but wild as in free."

"You know, when that dog got kilt at the Hippie House..."

Boss Lady cocked her head in question.

"The purple house," Sergeant Major said.

She nodded.

"That dog got kilt by some roving dogs. Tore it to pieces. They called out animal control. Those people said it could be Big Dog, but I told the officer no way would Big Dog do that."

Boss Lady replied that animal control had come to the farm and taken photos of Raven and Sweetie, but that she had never heard anything more about it.

Sergeant Major looked down at his shoes. "Really sorry Big Dog is gone," he said. "You gonna get another one?"

She stroked Sweetie's ears. "I don't think so..." Her voice trailed off. Sweetie wagged her tail.

The Sergeant Major got in his car and waved. Sweetie started to sing, and Boss Lady and the pack joined in.

* * *

Sweetie passed away in Boss Lady's arms, as Raven had two years before, at the farm with the vet. It was time. She could barely walk, and she had stopped eating and singing. She was buried beside Raven in a corner of the orchard by the old apple tree.

No more wolf-dogs were rescued or adopted by Boss Lady; the gravitational pull seemed to be toward herding dogs. But Raven and Sweetie had done what wolf-dogs do: reveal the wildness within us, the freedom to be who we are.

The Power of the Bark Side

A long time ago in a year far, far away…

Boss Lady and her best friend CeeCee, their two Oldenburg mares who were best friends, and their two dogs who were best friends, all went to Florida for the winter. It was January, 1990, when the Florida show circuit was still in its early stages, and the Wellington show grounds offered five vendors and a hot dog stand. The main arena was grass and spectators sat on the man-made swell to watch the competition. Boss Lady and CeeCee were going to Fox Lea Farm in Venice, Florida because their friends were there, and Fox Lea hosted a Concours Dressage International, or CDI—a competition recognized by the international horse sport organization known as the Federation Equestrian Internationale. CDIs hosted World Cup qualifying classes as well as, in certain years, Olympic and World Equestrian Games qualifying classes. It was an opportunity for both women to watch top horses and riders.

In the category of You-Can't-Make-This-Stuff-Up: when CeeCee and Boss Lady met, they discovered that they each had a dog they'd named after a Star Wars character. In human, nerdy Star Wars terms, this automatically made them soul sisters. The women also shared a penchant for giving their dogs an array of nicknames.

Princess Leia, also known as Leiah, Lei-Lei, Husky-Oatie, and Leia-Come was a Siberian husky/shepherd cross that had been dumped as an eight-week-old puppy onto the lawn of Robert E. Lee's birthplace where CeeCee was working. As a puppy, Leia consumed several pairs of shoes and a tennis racket. Several other personal items belonging to CeeCee disappeared during Leia's puppyhood, never to be seen again. Leia grew into a striking dog: wolf-grey with white legs and white face highlighted by the crown of black and grey that started at the top of her head like a widow's peak, and continued down the sides of her head and ears. Her prick ears were very prominent, like radar dishes that could pick up signals from Beijing. Those ears were always tuned in to something.

Wookie was a half Chow Chow, half Australian shepherd that Boss Lady rescued as an eight-week-old puppy. She was solid black except for a tiny white snip on her nose, and chest, and four white paws that looked like she was wearing sneakers. Her coat was that of a Chow: thick, black, double coated, with a tail that curled over her back. Her face, however, was all Australian shepherd: keen, almost fox-like, with ears that folded over like envelopes. She was known as The Wook, the Ninja Wook, Wookie-Come, and Wookie-No.

She earned her ninja name by blending into the night or hiding under a horse trailer to avoid being seen. Boss Lady could stand outside on a summer night and call Wookie ten times, not realizing the dog was ten feet away watching her from under a bush.

Wookie and Leia had traveled together during the fall show season. The first evening alone in the hotel room, Leia and Wookie had a party. They ripped the blinds off the window, scattered various toiletries, ate a bag of Doritos and threw the pillows around the room. When their humans returned from dinner it looked like the room had been ransacked. And there were Leia and Wookie, wagging their tails and barking their relief at their humans' safe return.

At a subsequent hotel stay, Wookie parked herself on top of the air conditioning unit, and parted the curtains with her paws and head so she could keep a watch out for her human's return. There was no room destruction, or even Dorito stealing. The key was for Wookie to be able to watch for her human.

On an early January morning in 1990, Boss Lady and CeeCee set out for Florida. Boss Lady drove a station wagon towing a tag-along camper, and CeeCee drove her truck and two-horse trailer. Angry Man had purchased two walkie-talkies for the women so that they could chatter the entire trip.

The trip started ominously when Boss Lady took a curve at too high a speed and the camper started to fishtail wildly, which caused the wires of the camper lights to break, leaving the camper with no signal lights or running lights.

They headed to Camden, South Carolina where they planned to spend the night. Hurricane Hugo had hit South Carolina and North Carolina just a few months earlier—a Category 4 hurricane—and as the women drove south, they saw the devastation: trees uprooted, pines broken like matchsticks.

In Camden they settled the mares into an old racehorse barn that a friend of Boss Lady's had suggested. All around the barn were the signs of the hurricane's force: trees empty of branches, fallen over as if a giant had clubbed every living arbor.

They fed the dogs in the hotel room (which had an air conditioning unit that Wookie could lie on), went out for dinner and then checked the horses.

In the morning they went back to the barn, let the dogs out to run around, and fed the horses. Once they got the horses on the trailer, they called for the dogs.

"Wookie come!"

"Leia come!"

Silence.

They called again.

One of the mares in the trailer stomped her foot with impatience, then kicked the ramp for good measure.

The women strained to hear something....paws crashing through the broken trees, a yip, a bark, a howl... nothing.

The swear words started to flow.

"Wookie come!"

"Leia come!"

The mare kicked the ramp again.

"We're going to have to take the horses off and go look for them," CeeCee said. Boss Lady tried to ignore the fear that they would never see their dogs again.

The women grabbed lead ropes and lowered the ramp. Suddenly they heard sounds on the slope of the woods, and there came Leia and Wookie, chasing each other through the fallen timber.

The dogs were quite pleased with themselves. They'd had a good run, smelled lots of interesting smells, and there was nothing like an adventure to make up for being leash-walked the night before. The women were relieved yet irritated. Humans can express both emotions in a way that is unique: "I am so glad to see you...don't ever do that again."

The trip continued uneventfully until Ocala, when the brakes on the camper decided to fail, making the action of stopping both station wagon and camper a combination of swear words and prayer.

They arrived in Venice Florida and took the horses off the trailer to discover that the bay mare had managed to pull two bales of hay out from under the hay feeder, kicked one bale under herself, and the other under her best friend. The next thing the women noticed is that the bay mare had pooped a pile of manure so high it looked like an elephant had been riding in the trailer. The other mare, who was CeeCee's, had just a few droppings. They walked the mares to the stalls, and then let the dogs out. The bay mare had a good roll in the new shavings, but CeeCee's mare, Wendemere, started to look uncomfortable.

Leia spotted a palm tree in the evening shadows and heard the rustling of the leaves. She planted herself there, gazing up to the top of the palm. Wookie ignored her and followed her own nose to the Cook Shack and the old food smells from a horse show weeks before.

The vet was called, the mare was oiled, given banamine, and two hours later began to eat. The dogs were corralled and the two exhausted women with their dogs gratefully retired to the camper.

At dawn's early light, Leia and Wookie begged, bounced, and howled their way out of the camper. As the women went to feed horses and unload gear from the trailer, the dogs went in search of the rustling sound in the palms....squirrels.

The squirrels could leap down the row of palm trees that marked the path between the shed row barns and the rings. Leia and Wookie chased the squirrels down the line of palms to the metal risers where spectators could sit to watch the rings. The squirrels would leap onto the risers, run across the top, and then leap onto a fence, climb another palm tree, and hurl abusive squirrel language at the dogs.

For Leia and Wookie, this was the ultimate cool-dog game: chase the squirrels from palm to palm, bark at the squirrels, try to climb up and catch the squirrels. The squirrels figured out that if they just stayed in the palm trees and didn't move, the chase was over. This new tactic puzzled Leia, but like her namesake character, she was not about to give up. She sat down at the bottom of a palm tree and looked up, never averting her gaze, in a classic coyote-and-moon pose.

Wookie had no such patience. She trotted off.

The women had just turned the mares out when someone came running to the barn yelling: "I think your dog is on Interstate 75!"

"Which dog?"

"The black one."

Boss Lady started running and yelling at the top of her lungs, "WOOKIECOME, WOOKIECOME, WOOKIECOME!"

Leia remained motionless under the palm tree. Surely, any minute now, the squirrel would make his move.

Boss Lady ran to the main barn and then into the wild palmetto jungle area, which was in the direction one of the riders had seen Wookie run. "I saw the dog on the shoulder of the interstate," someone called out.

"Watch out for snakes," another called out, and Boss Lady stopped dead in her tracks.

"WOOKIE COME!"

Real panic set in. Not your every-day-mild-anxiety-sky-is-falling panic: a full-range, nuclear panic fueled by the images of her dog trying to cross a busy interstate. She was trying not to cry, and instead chanted "ohmygod" twenty-five times in quick succession, while her body shook like a maraca, her brain needed a vacation from this emotionally stressful situation and drained itself of every single cell, leaving behind only the foggy remnants of the phrase "Wookiecome".

Another rider called out an offer to drive her to the interstate. Boss Lady nodded her head, grateful for the suggestion, and turned to follow the rider when suddenly the palmetto jungle parted and there came Wookie, panting and smiling, pleased as punch.

"What did I miss?' Wookie asked the Jack Russell terrier who barked at her.

"Your human is having a meltdown."

"WOOKIE!" Boss Lady hugged her, the brain cells that had gone AWOL slowly re-entered, set up shop, and began to repair synapses.

Wookie was not a heartless dog; when she saw her human, saw the panic and stress all over her face, Wookie vowed to herself she would not return to adventuring and scavenging for food along the interstate. She didn't tell Boss Lady this, and so was confined to a leash for 24 hours.

There was a routine to Florida life: Leia ran out every day to the first palm tree and sat looking up for the squirrel. Wookie patrolled the whole row of palm trees and the bleachers. If a squirrel made a move, the two dogs were on it, chasing the squirrel from palm tree to palm tree, back and forth, never tiring of the game.

While the dogs were on squirrel patrol, coffee was served in the camper. CeeCee was an excellent cook, and made a renowned pot of coffee, so friends came down from the main barn to have coffee, sit out at the picnic table and gossip before their first ride.

One of the morning coffee klatch regulars was Jon, a hairdresser from Canada, who had walked away from his lucrative hair-styling business and become a groom for a well-known dressage trainer. Jon would roar down to the shed row barn where CeeCee and Boss Lady were camped in his seasonal rental car from Rent-A-Wreck. It was a nondescript brown coupe with a tattered vinyl top whose loose strips fluttered like flags when he drove. One time he offered to take Boss Lady to the feed store and when she opened the passenger-side door, a host of Macdonald's burger wrappers, French fry containers, soda cans, half eaten potato chip bags, a crumpled Chips Ahoy bag, several beer bottles, and the well-worn pages of a paperback book by Dale Carnegie, *How to Stop Worrying and Start Living*, tumbled out of the car around her feet.

"Anything alive in here I need to know about?" she asked.

"Just some ants." He paused. "Regular ants, not fire ants."

"Nice of you to consider their wellbeing," she said, looking for a way to slide into the seat and not disturb any ants lingering under the Subway sandwich wrappers.

"We do what we can," he said.

With both passenger and driver windows rolled down, Jon threw the car into reverse, leaned as far back in the seat as he could, tilted his head back with both arms extended to the steering wheel, and yelled out the window, "Porsche. There is no substitute." Then he gunned the car down the sandy lane, vinyl roof strips flapping and several old hamburger wrappers on the ground in his wake.

In the afternoons, Wookie would head for the cool sand beneath the camper, out of the Florida sun. Leia rarely joined her, preferring the shady palms and squirrel patrol duties. Under the camper Wookie was virtually invisible, particularly when she tucked her paws underneath her. She enjoyed watching Boss Lady's feet move back and forth as she called her, and always waited to emerge until Boss Lady had turned her back and walked over to the shed row barn. Then Wookie would shed her invisibility, and crawl out into the sunlight.

In the evenings, the dogs hung around the picnic table as the humans ate dinner. Often, friends from the upper barn brought takeout or pizza and plenty of wine. Jon was always generous with pizza crust, slipping pieces under the table to the dogs. In the absence of television there were all sorts of games….Pictionary, Hollywood Gin Rummy, poker, and charades. A prominent Bermudian FEI rider, who went on to marry a Dutchman, live in Holland and compete in the

Olympics for Bermuda managed to win the most memorable night of charades with her rendition of Moby Dick—one which will remain in infamy.

CeeCee's boyfriend, Walter, arrived at Fox Lea Farm shortly after Boss lady and CeeCee had settled in. Walter had a German shepherd named JoJo.

Unlike Leia and Wookie, JoJo was attached to her owner like velcro. She literally never left his side. JoJo's ears, rather than standing straight up on either side of her head, actually formed a pyramid, the tops of her ears touching each other, giving the impression she was always listening. JoJo was the epitome of an obedient canine. It would not occur to her to take off running after squirrels without the full consent from her owner, in writing and notarized.

JoJo was not obedient out of fear, she was obedient out of love. Her human was nothing short of unique: Walter was an adventuresome Austrian, who thought nothing of hiking around India for a few months, traveling to the Himalayas, and then deciding to sell Austrian-crafted saddles in the US. Schedule, plans, a routine? Walter thought nothing of those things. He liked to let each day unfold like origami, holding his finger to the air to see in which direction his soul wanted to express itself that day. This kind of drove CeeCee crazy, and their arguments grew legendary as the season wore on. She was, after all, a dressage rider; precision, details, structure were her framework.

For JoJo, the only thing certain was that by late afternoon, Walter would head out to Sharky's bar on the beach to sit with CeeCee, drink beer, and watch the sun set over the ocean. JoJo would lie underneath his van, waiting patiently for him to return. Of course, Leia and Wookie tried to corrupt her, but JoJo had one mission in life: to take care of her wandering Austrian.

The farm hosted shows regularly—quarter horse shows, Appaloosa shows, dressage shows, hunter/jumper shows—and this was one of Wookie's most treasured times, because the Cook Shack would open to serve food to the visiting competitors. Wookie knew how to manipulate a human out of food. She sat up on her haunches with her front paws in front of her, cocked her head and stared. She could balance like this for quite a while until the human relented and gave her part of her egg salad sandwich or burger. Wookie trotted from picnic table to picnic table applying her trick. The few times she was utterly ignored by gossiping humans, she threw in her special trick: she flung herself on the ground, lay on her back with all four feet straight up in the air and laid very still. If a human said, "Look at that dog," or "That dog's playing dead," Wookie would leap to her feet, wag her tail, and sit up and beg for a potato chip. It never failed to get her free food.

Jon came running down to the shed row barn calling Boss Lady's name.

"Wookie's at the Cook Shack again and she's jumping on the picnic tables!"

Boss Lady ran with Jon to the Cook Shack and there was Wookie on top of one of the tables, begging. The riders were trying to get her off the picnic table, but in typical

Wookie fashion she was frozen in her sit-up mode, determined to get some sort of treat for her efforts.

"Wookie come!"

The dog did not move.

"I am so sorry," Boss Lady said to the riders as she approached the table.

Jon pulled a soggy, molasses-laden horse treat out of his pocket.

"Look what I have for you, Wook!" He held up the treat.

Wookie bounced off the table and was at his side in three seconds.

Leia looked over from her palm tree and said, "Woo woo, I want one, too."

The humans had a curious habit of giving nicknames to other riders, owners, horses, and dogs. The woman who, when asked how her ride went, always said, "like butter," became known as Mrs. Butter. The small group of junior riders who had come down to compete in the two-week Appaloosa circuit were known as "Children of the Corn" after their horses contracted ringworm and they didn't notify show management, thus exposing other horses who later stabled in those stalls to ringworm.

There was one husband of a trainer who gave himself his own nickname. He regularly flew down to Florida on the weekends, and then went back home to work during the week. One Monday morning he was headed to the airport with his brief case and Boss Lady saw him. There were three initials on his briefcase —"WTF"—and she asked what they stood for. He said without missing a beat, "What The Fuck," and so he became known as WTF, which was often shortened to WhatThe in polite company.

There was Peppermint Patty, Magilla in the Mist, Suzie Q, Daveed, Frick and Frack, and To and Fro. But there was one being on the farm named Winston (whom Jon called "the psycho dog from hell") who terrified every canine and nearly every human in the main barn—a dog so aggressive to other dogs and people, that his nickname became simply "Cujo". His owner made excuses for his behavior, and the upper barn dogs steered clear of him, even the Jack Russells. Riders would make a wide berth around Cujo even when he was tied up. And when the dog was let off his tether, all the upper barn dogs scattered and hid in tack rooms. Cujo was part Rottweiler, with a head that CeeCee called "wide as a dinner plate."

Leia and Wookie confined themselves to Palm Tree Squirrel Alley, the Cook Shack, and the bleachers. They had no interest in the upper barn, whether by instinct or basic disdain.

As the season wore on, the Cujo complaints from Jon, Susie Q, Peppermint Patty, and Daveed hung around the evening picnic table like fog. Nearly every day there was a new report about the dog's aggression, and he was venturing farther and farther out from the main barn to establish a larger territory.

One afternoon, CeeCee and Boss Lady were at the bleacher-end of the main arena just watching horses school. Jon was hand-walking a horse on the grass area by the ring. Wookie and Leia were lying in the shade after a serious game of squirrel tag. Suddenly, Cujo emerged from the barn and started coming towards the main arena.

Like a black bolt of lightning, Wookie took off towards Cujo. She moved faster than Boss Lady had ever seen.

"WOOKIE NO!"

Wookie hit Cujo full-force, knocking him over, and he screamed as he ran back to the barn, tail between his legs, shrieking in terror. Applause erupted from the main barn, as owners and riders and trainers all came out to see the terrifying Cujo reduced to squealing, running to his owner and cowering.

Wookie trotted back, and re-settled under the shade. Leia, not to be outdone, rolled one of the small Jack Russell terriers, who had come to see what the excitement was all about, and then strolled back to her place under the palms.

Cujo's reign of terror was over. His owner complained that he had been traumatized, but no one felt especially sorry for the dog that had chased and bullied the other dogs, and been aggressive toward the riders.

From that moment on, Wookie was officially christened: Bark Vader.

Spirit Dog

Spirit Dog was a blue merle Australian shepherd with two blue eyes that Boss Lady adopted from the local SPCA. He had been relinquished by his former owner because he kept running away. Spirit Dog zeroed in on Boss Lady the day she came to see him, and made his pronouncement by sitting on her feet, the Australian shepherd equivalent of "You are mine."

He was four years old when he came to the farm, and wasted no time in commandeering Boss Lady's bed and pillows, herding birds out of the boxwood bushes, and going on what Boss Lady called Spirit's Adventure Therapy, which included scoping out the neighbors, the main road, and the vast Western Virginia Paper Company timberland that bordered the farm.

When I arrived at the farm at the age of ten weeks, Spirit ignored me. He wasn't unpleasant, but just treated me as though as I was invisible. That still worked for me, because my whole world at that point was Boss Lady. Spirit and I started to pal around together when I was four months old. He was my mentor, teaching me all sorts of useful ideas such as: *blame it on the cats, water troughs are excellent cooling facilities,* and *obedience is overrated.*

Spirit did not much take to obedience, or rules in general. If the human said, "Spirit, come," he would consider the request, mull it over, examine his options, and then comply or not. Listening to the humans was always a choice, not an obligation. Boss Lady employed the treat-reward system, but Spirit was only mildly interested in bribes. If he felt the urge to go run through the forest, not even a filet mignon would change his mind.

He also liked to sing. His song was a *WooWooWu*, and he liked to sing it to our humans when he was feeling particularly affectionate. Boss Lady and Peter interpreted the *WooWooWu* as "I love you," and so they would say that to each other. Spirit would say, "See? You *can* teach humans new tricks."

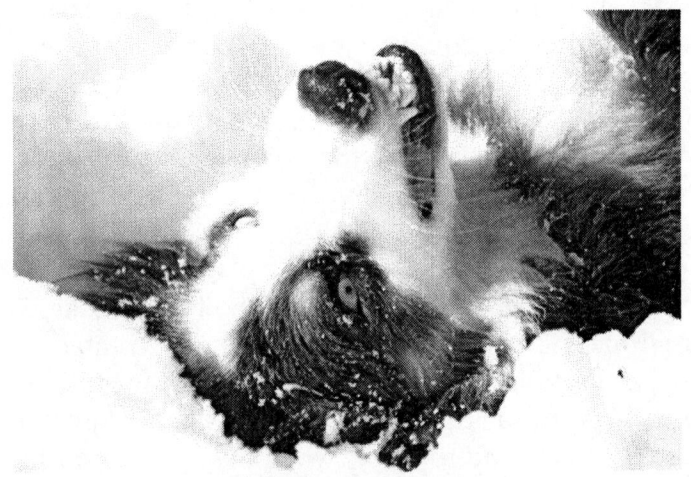

Spirit in the snow

As I grew up, Spirit looked for more ways to entertain himself, and to provide excellent Aussie protection. He chased off every hunting dog that put a paw on farm property, and began going down to the end of the driveway to sit there, guarding the entrance. For some reason he decided that he needed to guard from the middle of the road. He would stand on the pavement, while a car would come to a screeching halt to avoid hitting him. Even if they honked their horn, he wouldn't get out of the way.

One day Boss Lady was super-stressed, rushing around like a crazy woman. She threw the weekly bags of trash on the top of the Subaru and raced down the very long farm driveway to drop them in the trash container. She was so distracted that she forgot to stop and unload the green, bulging bags from the roof of the car. She also didn't notice that Spirit was galloping behind her. Off she went down the road, hitting a curve at Mach 1, driving like the proverbial bat out of hell. It wasn't until she careened into a gas station parking lot in town that she remembered she hadn't dumped the trash. She bounced out of the car and looked at the roof: empty.

Imagining a trail of garbage in her wake, she left the gas station and headed back to the farm. There were no signs of garbage remnants, and a panicky feeling in her escalated as the car climbed the hill to the farm driveway entrance. What had happened to the garbage? As she pulled up to the house, she had a fleeting thought that some good Samaritan had grabbed the garbage bags and disposed of them. She got out of the car and called Spirit.

There was an eerie silence except for the rescue dog, Jar Jar Binks, who barked that he was alive and well.

Boss Lady walked around the house, around the barn, and back down the driveway calling Spirit. Her heart started to beat a rhythm best suited for a rave concert. Then she jumped back into the car, leaving clouds of dust in her wake, pulled out into the road and drove slowly, calling Spirit's name.

And then she saw the garbage bags, there in a ditch by the road. And there, on closer inspection, was a blue merle Australian shepherd, lying comfortably in the ditch, guarding the garbage bags, and practicing his version of Zen meditation.

He opened his eyes and looked at her. *"What took you so long?"* he said as he stood up and walked calmly to the car.

* * *

Not long after his Guarding the Garbage Caper, Spirit was once again standing in the middle of the road when a truck came by and the driver stopped, thinking maybe this dog was lost. He had a collar but no tag, so the driver opened the door, Spirit jumped in, and off they went. Boss Lady, who had been at a funeral, drove up the driveway, let me out of the house, and called for Spirit. She walked around the barn calling him. She should have asked me. I already knew he was nowhere on the farm.

Boss Lady started to stress. A full-blown panic set in. She jumped in her car, and I jumped in with her to provide canine reassurance. She starting to drive like Richard Petty, whizzing out into the road, then slowing down to call his name: "Spirit! Spirit come!"
She drove a mile down the road, turned around and drove up the other direction, finally giving up and pulling into a

dirt logging road, rutted and not maintained. She got out of the car and called him, this time more like a plea than a command. She got back in the car, and started to back out of the logging road, but she didn't keep the car very straight, and the left rear tire veered into a ditch. Well, that resulted in a string of swear words that have probably never been uttered in that unique combination before.

Then she started to cry. There is nothing that tugs at a dog's heart strings more than feeling distress in our humans. I lurched up onto the middle console of the front seat and tried to lick her.

All of a sudden, a big four-wheel-drive truck pulled over next to the logging road. A man got out and approached the Subaru.

"I'm stuck" Boss Lady said, wiping her face with the back of her hand.

"Don't worry, ma'am, I've got tow cables, I can get you out."

"I was trying to find my dog," she said.

"What kinda dog were ya missin'?"

"He's an Australian shepherd, blue merle, two blue eyes."

The man leaned against the Subaru. "I know where your dog is. He's with my cousin, who lives on the corner down there at Route 616. Just came from his house."

"Oh my gosh, oh my gosh," Boss Lady blubbered, which was a little embarrassing for me, because normally she is quite eloquent.

The man pulled the Subaru out of the ditch. She offered to pay the man, who refused, and then she drove like Batman in the Batmobile several miles down to where the road dead- ended at Route 616. There on the corner was a big, red brick house with white pillars—a modern-day version of a plantation house. She had the good sense to drive relatively slowly down the paved driveway.

She knocked on the door. A woman opened it and Boss Lady blurted out, "Hi, I think you have my dog."

At that moment a man appeared next to the woman, an older gentleman, grey hair, very dapper.

"I ran into your cousin," Boss Lady said. "I mean, not literally, he helped me out of a ditch, and I told him I was looking for my dog, and he said you have him."

"What does your dog look like?" the man asked.

"He's an Australian shepherd, blue merle, two blue eyes."

"Yes, he is here," the man said, and opened the door to let Boss Lady in. "My wife gave him a bath."

The woman left the foyer and returned with a bathed and groomed Spirit at her side. "He's a lovely dog," the woman said.

Spirit, upon seeing Boss Lady, said, "WooWooWu" and ambled over to her and rubbed his head against her leg. "I had a nice time here, but I'm ready to go home," he said.

"Found him standing in the middle of the road," the man said.

"He didn't have a tag," the woman said.

"I know," Boss Lady said. "He keeps losing his name tags. They fall off his collar."

"He could have been hurt out there in the road," the man said.

"I know," Boss Lady sighed. "But he feels his job is to guard the entrance to the farm."

Spirit happily trotted out to the car with Boss Lady. I was ecstatic to see him. But he didn't smell like himself. He smelled like a perfume bottle.

"First thing I'm gonna do when we get back to the farm," Spirit intimated, "is roll in horse manure and maybe rendezvous with a skunk."

* * *

For two months, Spirit did not wander, did not go to the end of the driveway, did not play chicken with cars on the road. Then one December morning when I was eleven months old, we were outside before sunrise, enjoying the cold air, and Spirit picked up the scent of deer. When he saw the does, he took off after them with me in pursuit, running over the frozen ground. It was exhilarating!

The deer ran into a tree line that bordered the road, bounded across the road, with Spirit and me behind them.

I never saw the car. I never heard the car. And maybe the car didn't see me, but it collided with me, and the impact sent me tumbling into the roadside ditch. I found myself unable to move. My left hip was broken. The car never stopped.

Spirit headed home. When Boss Lady saw him without me, she started searching the woods, the fields, calling my name. Spirit was with her, and kept trying to point with his head the direction of the ditch that I lay in. She didn't get it.

Lucky for me, the neighbors living across from the ditch I lay in saw me and called animal control, who came, read my name tag, and called Boss Lady who, just as I knew she would, came roaring up the hill from the driveway like she was coming to the finish line of the Indy 500.

I was so glad to see her! The animal control officer picked me up and put me in the Subaru, and Boss Lady speed-dialed the vet while chanting, "Please be okay, please be okay, please be okay."

I ended up having to go to an orthopedic specialist outside of Richmond, where I had surgery, got pinned and screwed, and
spent a week in the hospital. It wasn't too bad; the vet techs loved me. I figured out when I was a wee pup that

schmoozing the vet techs got me extra treats and special attention. It is a philosophy I have embraced my entire life.

* * *

Following the deer episode, Spirit stayed on the farm. He had no desire to head down the drive, or to have any adventure therapy. It was as if the wanderlust had just disappeared. That lasted a year.

He was standing in the road on an autumn afternoon when a car slowed down and then stopped, flashers on. Spirit stood there, curious, but not curious enough to move. A young woman got out of the car, came over to him and asked, "Are you lost, Doggie?"

"No, I am not lost. I live right here." He looked towards the driveway and the farm sign.

"You poor dog," she said, and petted him. She felt his collar but there were no tags. "Come with me, Doggie, we'll find your home."

She opened the car door, and naturally Spirit jumped in. Going for car rides was always one of his favorite forms of travel. He especially liked riding in the bed of the farm truck as the wind whistled through his coat.

The woman talked to him as she drove. He enjoyed her back seat, although it was smaller than the Subaru's. What he liked best about being in the back seat was the feeling of being in a limousine, driven by his own personal chauffeur. He guessed she was taking him to her house where she'd probably feed him, and he was fine with that. The car finally stopped and the woman turned off the ignition.

"Here we are," she said. She took a belt from around her jeans and attached it to his collar.

As soon as he was out of the car he realized he had been at this place before. It was the SPCA, where he had met Boss Lady when he had been surrendered. The woman talked to a man inside the building. A slip lead was put over Spirit's head, and he was led back to the cages.

Meanwhile, Boss Lady and I were at a horse show, out of state. It was a phone call from Peter that alerted Boss Lady to Spirit being AWOL. She reminded Peter to drive up and down the road and call for him, and of the people in the big house who took him in before. All this was done, and there was no Spirit.

Take a woman who is away from home and hears her dog is missing, and let me tell you…it isn't pretty. After instructing Peter to go check with the neighbors, make signs, and call the SPCA, she proceeded to cling to me like I was a teddy bear, and I was happy to oblige, but the pacing, the wringing of the hands, and the frequent mantra—"Where the hell IS he?"—was a little over the top.

The following morning, after Boss Lady had spent most of the night imagining she had lost Spirit forever, Peter called. The SPCA had Spirit, and he was on his way to get him.

She danced around that hotel room. She made me dance with her. She gave me treats just for being me. Of course, I had known all along that Spirit was okay. We dogs know these things.

Peter called her when he had Spirit safely in his truck.

"Does he look okay?" Boss Lady asked. "How is he?"

Peter started to chuckle. "Well, Spirit managed to con the volunteers into letting him hang out with them in the reception area. There he was, lying beside the desk being fawned over when I got there."

"You mean he wasn't in one of those cages in the dog wing?"

"Oh, no, he evidently got to spend the night up in one of the offices with a dog bed. He is a true canine con artist. You know, the special prisoner—the celebrity who can't be in with the rest of the prison population."

From that moment on Peter referred to him as Jailbird, a moniker Spirit actually enjoyed. It sounded dangerous and cool at the same time. He was very appreciative of Peter for his rescue, and often spoke of him to the pack as The Guy Who Sprung Me from the Big House.

After his night in the clink, Spirit decided to stick around the farm. He got a new collar with his name and Boss Lady's phone number engraved on an attached brass plate. But eventually that wanderlust would take hold again, and he'd be off on what he called a "mini-adventure". He no longer stood in the middle of the road.

Unlike me, Spirit was not competitive. I loved to launch myself off the bank into the pond to catch a Frisbee, but Spirit preferred swimming languidly around the pond like an alligator, just his nose and the top of his head above the water. If Peter threw a stick or a ball, I was on it, but Spirit just kind of yawned at the whole idea... "You actually want me to get that stupid stick and bring it back?" Then he would lie down on the ground and roll over onto his back with all four feet in the air, punctuating his opinion of fetching.

* * *

One night he suffered a kind of a stroke, or what some might call a neurological event. He recovered, but had spatial distortion problems. He slowed down quite a bit, and spent a lot of time resting. His appetite was good, but he ate slowly, lying on the floor with the bowl between his paws. I wondered if he did that on purpose, as we had to stand around and watch him eat.

"Yum," he would say to me, and take another bite, after I had gobbled up my food and licked the bowl with the speed of lightning.

One morning, he started bumping into things, becoming very anxious and distressed. Then he fell over and couldn't get up. Peter carried him to the car, and I jumped in too for company. Boss Lady careened into the vet clinic lot, and the techs took Spirit out of the car on a stretcher.

I knew. And Boss Lady knew.

I laid on the floor beside Spirit with Boss Lady next to us. The vet said something about a brain tumor.

Spirit whispered, "Don't let me suffer. I'm ready."

As Boss Lady held his head in her lap, I spoke to him, thanked him, watched and waited for his soul to leave. As soon as it did, I would not look at him again. Spirit was no longer in that body; it was an empty shell. Both the vet and Boss Lady registered my reaction, the turn of my head away from the canine form on the floor. It wasn't my friend Spirit. He had already left the building.

Boss Lady and Peter grieved for a long time. In a way they are still grieving, but it is no longer painful. They remind each other of funny Spirit stories, and a photograph of him in the snow sits in a prominent place. Every night, when Boss Lady turns out the lights in the living room, she looks at that photo of Spirit and says goodnight to him.

Spirit is the reason I am with Boss Lady. Spirit is the reason Thunderbear, Buckaroo, and Crockett are with Boss Lady. Spirit was the Australian shepherd whose personality drove her to fall in love with the breed.

When Spirit passed, I became the Boss Dog, the Big Kahuna, the Storyteller of the Tribe. He lives on in the stories I tell of him to the younger pack members, as he lives on in the reminiscences of our humans. I heard Boss Lady tell Peter one day, when she got all teary-eyed about Spirit, "I wouldn't trade one tear if it meant never having a Spirit Dog in my life."

The way I see it, if Spirit Dog has not reincarnated into a different type of body—some kind of Buddhist anarchist monk or a charismatic mastermind à la *Ocean's Eleven*—then I imagine I will see him gliding along in a pond like an alligator, sleeping under the trees on his back with all four feet in the air, or wandering off in search of adventure in that interdimensional place after death. I imagine he will greet me when I get there, and we'll have a good run together through the fields, and then I will tell him the stories of those I left behind.

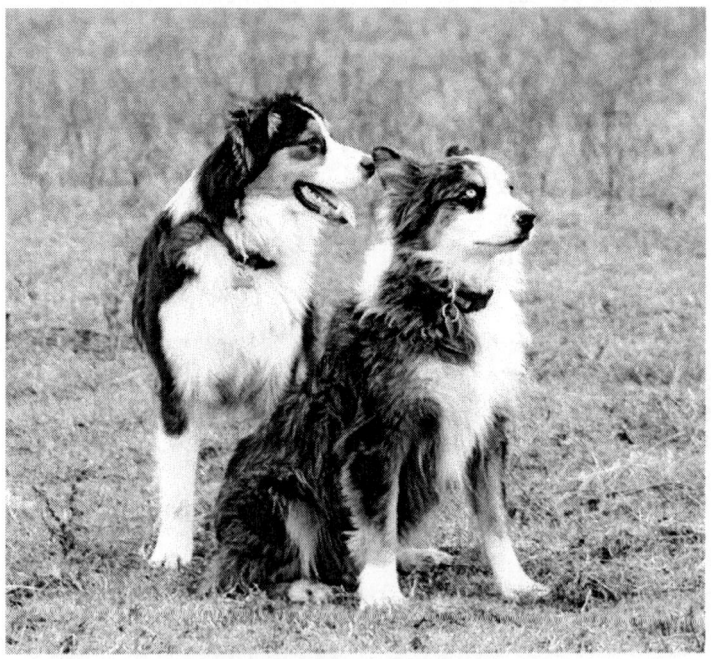

Kemosabe and Spirit Dog

Fowl Play

Chickens are unusual creatures. They are avians and mini-dinosaurs rolled into one. Any dog that lives with chickens and who has sat through *Jurassic Park* on TV knows that having chickens around is akin to living with miniaturized Velociraptors and T. Rexes.

They eat anything. They will try to take marrow bones from members of the dog pack. They consider bison and fish a delicacy. They slurp leftover bone broth, lentil soup, and the last remaining contents of the kefir bottle. They will attack a row of kale and consume it within minutes, leaving the poor stalks bare, then move on to the lettuce, radish greens, and beet tops.

The job of the dog pack is to keep the chickens from ransacking the garden. This is a delicate job, because chickens actually serve a purpose in a garden: they aerate the soil. However, the humans like the soil aerated after the harvest, before the cover crops and manure are laid down. Chickens don't understand this. They think they have the right to parade into any area on the farm, take their dirt baths, and eat every insect and vegetable offering in sight. They also like to go into the horse stalls, make a nest, lay eggs, fluff up the straw and redistribute it. Boss Lady gets annoyed when she has just bedded a stall, and comes back to find the chickens have rearranged it.

That's where the pack comes in. We take it upon ourselves to drive those pesky little dinosaurs out of the garden, and out of the stalls. Ideally, of course, we would wait for our humans to tell us when to move the chickens. Sometimes we are too enthusiastic. Buckaroo has landed on more than one hen, which is a little bit like an NFL fullback landing on a chickadee. The hens have managed to survive without injury, probably because all his hair made the impact a little softer.

Egg-stealing is another pastime enjoyed by the pack. Of course, it's easy to grab an egg from a nest in a stall, but it takes more sheer athleticism to get an egg from a nest in the top of the hay stack. The absolute best egg-stealing happens when the human has been to the chicken house, collected the eggs, and then sets the basket down to fill water bowls for chickens. With her back turned, one or more of the pack will grab an egg and find a nice place to lie down and eat it. Sometimes the human remembers to tell us, "Leave it," and we obligingly obey... except for yours truly. Sneaking an egg is a great game of skill and timing. I am excellent at it.

Sometimes the pack enjoys playing Scatter the Dinos. This entails running full-speed into a group of chickens under one of the boxwood bushes. They squawk, fly into the air, and scatter like plump dumplings. Thunderbear is the master at this game because he is fast and light-footed, and the chickens don't hear him coming.

At one time, there was a group of eight hens on the farm known as The Ladies. They were a Rhode Island Red cross and had arrived together as pullets. They always moved around the farm in a group, cackling to each other like women having lunch at a deli. They were also adventurous. Any open door was investigated, including those of the house, cars, trucks, and horse trailers. When a fence contractor came to put up new fences, several of the hens hopped into one of the trucks with a door open, and got into the man's lunch. They thought his ham sandwich was most excellent. On another day, one of them flew up into the back of the Subaru when the tailgate was open and the human was taking groceries out. Boss Lady had just walked into the house with some bags, and the chicken flew up into the car and started pecking around the roast, which was going to be dog food that night.

On a very windy, cold, October afternoon, after the humans had started a fire in the fireplace, the chimney started roaring and a spark caught in a chink in the old slate roof, starting a roof fire, fanned by the wind.

There are certain kinds of crises that Boss Lady is adept at handling: horse injuries, colic, dog bit by poisonous snake, injuries to other humans. But a fire on the roof is not in her wheelhouse of crisis management. She freaked out.

"PETER! PETER!" she yelled at the top of her lungs as she fumbled with her cell phone to call 9-1-1, visions of the entire roof exploding in flames running through her head. She drove the pack out of the house, and grabbed the two cats, who were clearly annoyed and agreed between themselves to report her as in violation of the Geneva Convention ruling on the transportation of felines from couch to cold, windy terrace, with no can of tuna in sight.

Peter sprinted out of the barn where he had been working. Boss Lady was babbling into the phone to the 9-1-1 operator and pointing to the roof. Peter grabbed a chair, a ladder, and somehow shimmied up the porch roof and then inched his way up the steep pitch of the slate roof like Spider-Man. Boss Lady stood below chanting, "Ohmygod, ohmygod, ohmygod". Sparks were flying from the ongoing chimney fire.

"Get me water!" Peter yelled.

She stood like a statue, as if her feet were frozen to the ground, while her mind spun possibilities: *Go to the barn and get a bucket? Go into the house and get a pot of water?*

"The spigot right there," Peter called down. "With the hose attached. Turn it on and pass it up to me."

She leaped into action, now that it didn't require thinking, turned on the hose, and looked up at Peter. He slid down the roof, stopping his forward momentum by jamming his foot into the gutter. On sheer willpower and adrenalin, he leaned down and she threw the hose up towards him. The water hit his face, but he didn't care; he had the hose and was now crawling back up the roof to get to the fire.

"Put the fire out in the fireplace," he yelled.

She ran into the house where the roar of the chimney had receded, filled pots with water and threw it on the fire. Then she heard the sounds of the fire trucks.

Men in firefighter gear poured out of trucks. Some were walking up the long drive hauling hoses from the trucks parked at the farm drive entrance. The pack barked the alarm, as Spirit Dog was convinced aliens had landed. A fireman ran up to the house and looked at Peter up on the roof.

"Let us get you down, sir."

"The fire's out," Peter said, spraying another part of the roof with water just to be sure.

Boss Lady came running out of the house, vibrating like a whirligig. An official looking man got out of his car and introduced himself as an assistant fire chief as more firemen walked up the driveway—two fire companies in all.

They threw up a big ladder, and a fireman helped Peter down, and then two firefighters got up on the roof, while three more went into the house, checked the fireplace, went up into the second floor, hacked out some ceiling to make sure no fire was lurking, while the firemen on the roof pulled up slates, looking for more burning sparks.

The pack had quieted down and was focused on marking the left tires of the trucks with a message: Property of the Pack.

Firemen stood in groups, discussing the roof, the chimney, the wind direction. Boss Lady had finally reached a degree of calm; all the animals were safe, and the house had not burned down.

Suddenly from around the corner of the house came the Ladies, marching onto the front lawn now that the commotion had passed, to see if there were any tidbits of food among the broken roof slates and burned pieces of wood. Several firemen gasped and pointed to the flock, as one young fireman mumbled, "What the hell?"

Chickens appearing after a fire evidently is not a common occurrence when a fireman's experience is with fires fought in suburban neighborhoods and city buildings.

"Oh, that's just the Ladies," Boss Lady explained.

The flock spread out, pecking around the heavy rubber boots of the firemen as if they were roots of trees. A couple of firemen moved quickly away from the pecking beaks, a sure indication that the chicken they were accustomed to, wrapped in plastic at the grocery store, didn't normally move around and cluck. The hens moved in a kind of fearless consciousness, undaunted by hoses, ladders, or the humans on the roof securing a tarp over the hole. One hen tried to fly onto one of the fire trucks to get a better view, missed the landing spot, and on her second attempt managed to land on the hood, whereupon she informed the rest of the flock that despite the view, there were no edibles.

"Those aren't chickens," the assistant fire chief said, as several hens pecked around the roof debris. "Those are warriors."

Henceforth, the Ladies became known as the Warrior Chickens.

Long before the Warrior Chickens came to the farm, when Boss Lady was married to Angry Man, they bought six Pekin ducklings and two young turkeys.

The ducklings were named after political figures: Ross Perot, Barbara Bush, George Bush, Bill Clinton, Hillary Clinton, and Nancy Reagan. Boss Lady named the turkeys Anthony and Cleopatra, but Angry Man referred to them as Thanksgiving and Christmas...meaning dinner.

Bear Dog was a Labrador/German shepherd mix Boss Lady had adopted from the SPCA when he was ten weeks old. Other than some tan points on his legs, cheeks, and under his eyes, and a rather bushy tail, he looked like a black Labrador. His tail rarely stopped wagging, and he could sweep contents off the coffee table in nanoseconds.

Boss Lady called him The Happy Dog, because Bear was so good- natured and easy-going. That is, until the ducks arrived...

The ducklings were eight weeks old when they were given some freedom to forage beyond their duck enclosure. Ross Perot was the first one Bear took down, followed in quick succession by George and Barbara—all within the space of five minutes.

Bear dog didn't eat them. He carried each body faithfully to the back door and dropped it there.

Naturally, this caused great concern from the humans, who loved Bear Dog, but also wanted to raise the ducks. So Angry Man tied a dead duck around Bear Dog's neck, and locked him up in the duck enclosure with the surviving ducks.

Those young ducks quacked at that dog until they were hoarse. Bear Dog sat in misery in the middle of the enclosure with the dead duck around his neck, while the rest of the ducks called him rude names in duck-speak that are not appropriate in present company.

Bear Dog never so much as looked at another duck again.

The ducks became known as the Quackers. Hillary Clinton Quacker outlived Bill Clinton Quacker when a fox ran off with him. She and the other remaining duck, Nancy Reagan Quacker, developed a particular penchant for chasing dogs, raiding and plundering tomatoes from the garden, and following the humans on walks around the farm.

The turkeys were lovingly cared for by Boss Lady, who diligently tried to speak turkey. Angry Man wanted to eat Anthony and Cleopatra, but Boss Lady considered them pets. She managed to keep them alive during Thanksgiving, but as his rage at not getting his way escalated as Christmas day neared, she was unable to save Anthony from the dinner table.

A friend who was visiting from West Virginia for the holidays prepared the bird, basted it, and cooked it. When the turkey came out of the oven, Boss Lady ran out of the kitchen overcome by waves of nausea.

"If you were starving, you'd eat it," Angry man said.

"Well, I am not starving and I am not going to eat Anthony."

"Never name 'em," the friend said. "Don't name anything you plan on eatin'."

Cleopatra was found in her enclosure dead of unknown causes a month after Anthony became Christmas dinner. Boss Lady was convinced she died of a broken heart.

* * *

The dog pack is entrusted with protection of the chickens. However, there is a lineage of red foxes on this farm that outsmarts the pack in very unusual ways.

The Son of a Son of The Big Red Fox carries on raids in the middle of a hot summer afternoon. When the canines are resting in the shade, or hanging out in the air conditioning, this lineage of The Big Red Fox will sit in the middle of the driveway, sizing up opportunity. Peter has watched the fox slip by a sleeping Australian shepherd on its way to try to intercept a chicken pecking away at birdseed that has fallen from a feeder.

What the humans don't know is that the Son of a Son of The Big Red Fox has, on more than one occasion, uttered the fox equivalent of *neener neener neener* to one or more of the pack members when we have spotted him in tall grass. He's a quick little bugger, and as fast as Crockett is, even he can never catch him.

Peter set up a Havahart trap when the raids became more daring. That fox looked at the trap with the tasty meat inside and burst out laughing. The only creatures the trap caught were ants.

After that, the new strategy was a kind of truce between human and fox—or as I like to call it, "The Humans Said Uncle". Peter, who has a particular affinity for foxes, stood on the edge of the woods and proclaimed that the fox could share the chickens with the humans as long as the entire flock was not decimated. Thunderbear said it was a lot like being on a sinking ship and asking the sharks to not eat all the sailors.

Funny thing, though... the fox raids stopped. At first Peter thought the fox had been shot or run over. Months passed and no sign of the little red demon. Fall turned into winter, no fox. Then spring arrived, and who should come trotting up the driveway but the Son of a Son of The Big Red Fox.

We saw him and gave chase. Buckaroo called out to the fox as we ran: "Planning on chicken take-out?" The fox crossed into the woods and down towards the pond, and we raced after him. Little did we know that his vixen was under the old hay barn. While we galloped off to chase her mate, she calmly sneaked up to the house, grabbed a hen, and left a trail of feathers in her wake.

So Peter decided the flock needed a rooster. He bought a young rooster from a boy who had raised him from a chick and called him Sweetie—admittedly a strange name for a rooster, but Peter kept it. This rooster looked like he stepped out of a 19th-century English painting. The hens at first thought he was the male equivalent of Typhoid Mary. He was shunned, ignored, pecked, and thoroughly emasculated. He endured this treatment until he developed the chicken equivalent of *cojones*. Then he began to boss the hens around, choose his favorites, and in typical male fashion, started to run the show. He also liked to have sex multiple times per day with various hens, but did not yet produce any offspring. As Boss Lady says, "he's shooting blanks."

Make no mistake, that rooster is not one to trifle with. He tries to chest bump Buckaroo and Crockett if they get into his personal space, and one time challenged a red-tailed hawk, who gave up and flew away. But he really earned his rank as mini-T. Rex when he took on the fox.

The Son of a Son of The Big Red Fox was hiding under the horse trailer as the hens were settling down under the boxwoods and the humans were out by the barn working in the garden. Suddenly the mini-T. Rex sounded the alarm, puffed himself up to twice his size and took on that fox with his wings, spurs, and beak. The pack came running and the fox exited left, sending us on a good long run that ended with the fox diving into his burrow. Thunderbear did try to dig him out, but the excavation process was too big an undertaking, and besides, our effort at running the fox off was worth getting back to the humans and having some treats.

The irritating part about living with a rooster who successfully defends his flock from predators is that the rooster walks around crowing, "Yo, I'm the man," when we all know that it would be "Yo, I'm the fried chicken" if he didn't live on a farm owned by vegetarians.

Tigger Montague

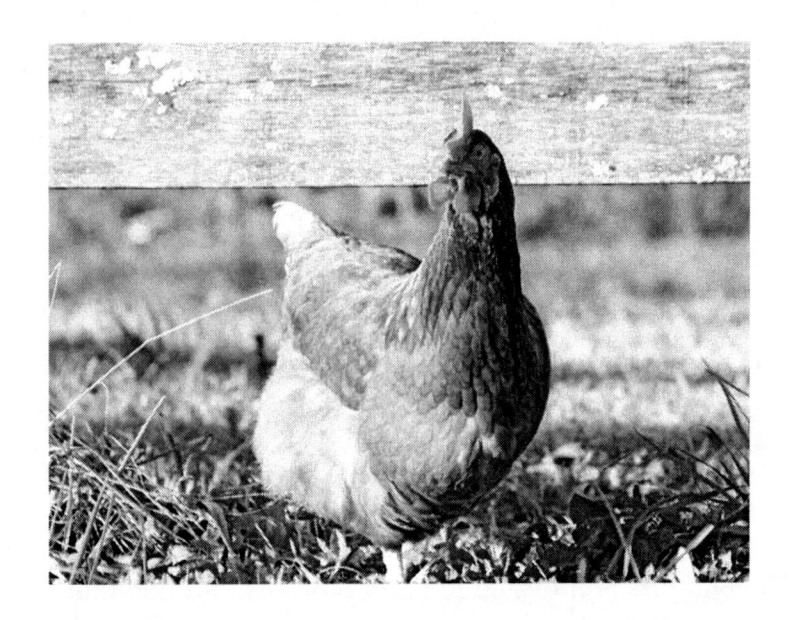

I Herd You

The American Kennel Club has divided dog breeds into groups: Hound, Working, Sporting, Terrier, and Toy. There is also the Non-Sporting Group, which is a varied collection of breeds such as poodle, bulldog, bichon, Dalmation, Lhasa apso and shiba inu. Then there is the Herding Group, the newest group in the AKC, formed in 1983 from breeds that were originally in the Working Group.

For some reason that is not exactly clear, Boss Lady loves herding dogs, probably because herding dogs are a lot like she is: driven, bossy, and competitive. The fact that one of the family dogs from her childhood was a border collie might explain a little of her attraction to herding dogs.

Her youngest brother named the border collie "Spike" for reasons unknown. Spike had no sheep or cattle or horses to herd, so he herded the children. He thought bicycles and tricycles needed his immediate reprimand, and often bit their tires as the children rode in the driveway, causing innumerable falls and wails of, "Bad Spikey!"

Boss Lady's parents appreciated Spike's protective instincts when it came to teenage boys coming to hang out with Boss Lady or take her out on a date. The dog would place himself between Boss Lady and the young man, running interference if the young man got too close to her on the couch. Spike would jump up to be between them, nip ankles, or start the ever-reliable barking to alert the parents that there was some *funny business* going on in the den.

The beginnings of Boss Lady's adult passion for herding dogs began with two red corgis named Kizzie and Toby. Kizzie was short for "Kismet" and Toby was given his name by his breeder. The fact that both names are actually characters in the *Roots* TV miniseries was purely accidental.

Toby's coat was the color of an egg yolk (the deep, rich color of a local, organic, free-range chicken egg yolk—not the pale, anemic color of a store-bought egg), hence he was known as Toby the Egg.

He was a most excellent excavator, digging holes that fit his long body up to the shoulders, but with enough room that his head and paws could comfortably lie on the surface, so that he was three-quarters submerged. Digging the right hole meant excavating many small holes before finally getting it just right. The smaller, abandoned holes were perfect for tripping unsuspecting humans and twisting ankles. Every hole that was covered up was subsequently re-dug by Toby. Never underestimate a corgi's determination.

Kizzie was the herder. She was the runt of her litter and she was small, but agile and quick. She was especially fond of herding cats. She wasn't a cat chaser, she simply like to drive the cats to what she considered appropriate cat places: in the shower stall, outside through the cat door, and onto the porch. She thought furniture belonged to the dogs, as well as specific areas of the house: living room, kitchen, dining room, and bedroom.

This did not sit well with one of the resident cats, King Henry of Springdale. King Henry was a big, long-haired, grey cat with four white paws, including two front ones the size of catcher's mitts. Had he been in human form, he would have joined a motorcycle gang, worn a black leather jacket, had numerous tattoos, and smoked cigarettes. Boss Lady had rescued him from the SPCA when he called out to her that he was being held prisoner. Naturally she adopted him.

King Henry didn't think much of being herded by a corgi. It was a basic assault on his principles of catdom: *dogs have masters, cats have staff.*

Every time Kizzie tried to herd King Henry by walking behind him with her nose at the level of his hind leg hocks, he'd abruptly stop, whirl around and box her face. Those catcher's-mitt paws of his could carry quite a punch, even with the claws retracted. Kizzie would yip, back up, and as soon as he started sauntering again, she was nose-to-hock with his back legs.

It was a quiet, lazy, summer afternoon and King Henry had commandeered one of the floor vents, which puffed his white belly hair as the air conditioning unit cycled. He was hungry, and it was time for an afternoon snack, the second lunch of the day. He stood up, stretched, glanced at the sleeping corgis on the couch, and ambled towards the kitchen. Suddenly Kizzie was awake and flying off the couch. Toby lifted his head from one of the pillows, saw the grey cat's body with his tail in the air, and Kizzie behind him in her herding mode, decided time was better spent sleeping.

Kizzie moved to the right side of the big cat to block him from getting to the cat food and hopefully divert him out the cat door. The cat was not to be deterred. He managed to twist his body around, swinging his haunches by pivoting on his front feet so that he was now in front of Kizzie. He stood up on his hind legs, boxed her a few times, then hissed and spit for good measure. The corgi backpedaled from the flying boxer paws, and the cat continued: a right hook, a left hook, pursuing her into the living room. Kizzie turned from her pursuer. The cat extended one set of paw claws and swiped her on the fanny. She yelped, she cried, she launched herself onto the safety of the couch. The cat sat down and cleaned his paws, as doggie residue is a known contaminant, and after his paws were satisfactorily clean, made his way slowly to the kitchen and the food bowls.

Never underestimate the lengths a cat will go to when it wants a snack.

Rocky Raccoon was a blue heeler, also known as an Australian cattle dog. He had been bred by a local farrier, who raised the litter of puppies in an old horse trailer. Rocky was only nine weeks old when the farrier, called out for an emergency shoeing on a horse who had lost a shoe during a dressage clinic, came to the barn with the little puppy. Rocky looked like a raccoon, the black mask around his eyes highlighted by copper-brown markings around it. He had a fluffy coat not within the standard of the breed. He also had a Siberian husky-like tail that curled up over his back. He was shy; it was his first time away from the other puppies and the only human he knew was the farrier.

The clinic riders picked him up and carried him around, but it was Boss Lady who fell in love with him. He sat on her lap and didn't move.

The clinician, a Dutchman, teased Boss Lady about the puppy. "Do you know how to say no?" he asked her, but it was pointless. When a human falls for a dog, there is no antidote. On the spot, she named him Rocky Raccoon. Naturally, the Beatles song of the same name was something she sang to him on a daily basis.

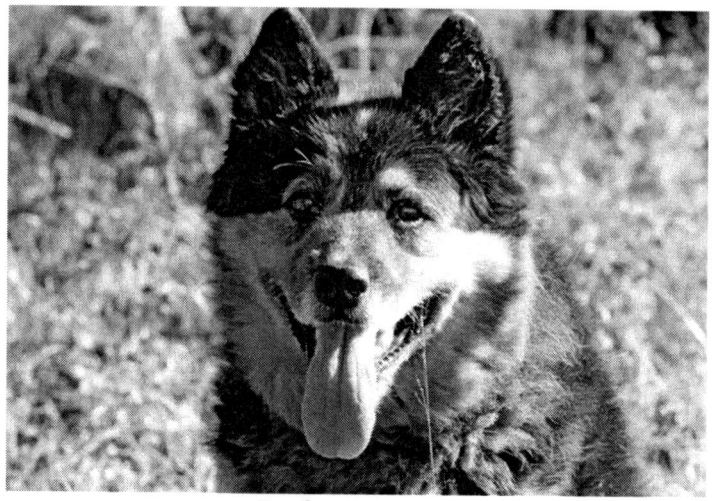

Rocky Raccoon

Rocky had an obsessive talent: catching things. It could be a Frisbee, a ball, a stick, a shoe, even a blade of grass. Throw it and he would catch it, bring it right back and drop it in your lap or at your feet. Boss Lady said she never taught him this. He just did it on his own, starting when he was just a few months old and she threw him a stuffed toy, which he promptly brought back to her. He lived to catch and retrieve.

At horse shows, he would bring a glove, a sock, or a piece of hay or straw and drop it at a human's feet, then stand back, wag his tail, crouch low and wait. If the human did nothing, he would pick up the piece of hay and drop it again. He would repeat this until the piece of hay was thrown. Now, pieces of hay don't fly very far, but he didn't care. With the short flight distance, he would either catch it in mid-air or pounce on it and immediately bring it back.

If Boss Lady was busy, he would trot down the barn aisle to find a human sitting outside her stall, and he would bring her the piece of hay or straw and wait until she threw it. Certain humans did not appreciate Rocky's gift of slobbery hay in their lap, which often left a telltale green slime residue on their newly washed, white show breeches.

Rocky's relentless pursuit of catching and retrieving did get him into trouble on more than one occasion. He never learned the word "stop". This became an issue when a man decided to throw Rocky a Frisbee on one of the hottest and most humid days of the year—because Rocky, no matter how far the Frisbee flew or how high, gave it his all. He was quite adept at catching the Frisbee in mid-air using his athleticism to launch himself skyward.

On this very hot, humid day with temperature in the mid-90s and a heat index of 100, Carl, a friend of one of the grooms, was visiting the training barn where Boss Lady kept her horse. She had taken her horse into the indoor arena for some light work, leaving Rocky in the stable. Rocky brought the man his Frisbee, which the man threw and threw and threw, utterly unaware of how dangerously hot the dog was getting. Of course, Rocky would not stop of his own volition.

When Boss Lady came into the barn from the indoor, she saw the man throwing the Frisbee to Rocky, who was exhausted, but still trying to run to catch it. Horrified, she grabbed Rocky, who was panting so hard she was afraid he was going to get heatstroke. She put him in the wash stall and started running water on him. He was having a hard time catching his breath, and his tongue was three times its normal size. She focused the hose on his head, neck and between his legs. He lay down in the wash stall, lapping up the spilled water a little at a time.

"You can't throw a Frisbee for thirty minutes in this weather!" she snapped at Carl, who stood there helplessly.

"I thought he would stop if he got too hot," Carl said.

"This dog wouldn't stop even if he only had one leg! I just can't believe you couldn't see his distress."

"Ignorant," one of the riders murmured.

"Thinks a dog like Rocky is some kind of machine," another rider said.

"Maybe you need to throw the Frisbee to Carl for thirty minutes in this weather," a third rider piped up.

Carl slunk out to his car. Never underestimate female dressage riders and their ability to perform a vasectomy with words.

Luckily, Rocky made a quick recovery after spending some time in the air-conditioned riders' lounge. To no one's surprise, he was back in the barn looking for his Frisbee.

Rocky went everywhere with Boss Lady. He never needed a leash, he just stayed right by her side. He loved to get in the bed of the big dually truck for the weekly trip to the feed store. Once, he jumped out of the bed as she was in the store paying for feed. The men were loading the feed onto the truck and Rocky was trying to get them to throw him something. Boss Lady came out of the store and got in the cab, never looking at the bed of the truck. She drove home, got out of the cab, and realized: no Rocky Raccoon. She called the feed store, and yes, Rocky was there, sitting by the entrance waiting for her.

He went to horse shows, the hardware store, the UPS shipping store. He even went a few times to Dulles Airport when Boss Lady had to pick up the Dutch clinician who flew in every few months to give a dressage clinic. He stayed in motels, hotels, and enjoyed outside patios at restaurants in the summer. He was particularly popular with the owner of the local Subaru dealership, who loved having Rocky visit when Boss Lady's car was in for service. As the owner said, "That's the smartest dog I ever saw."

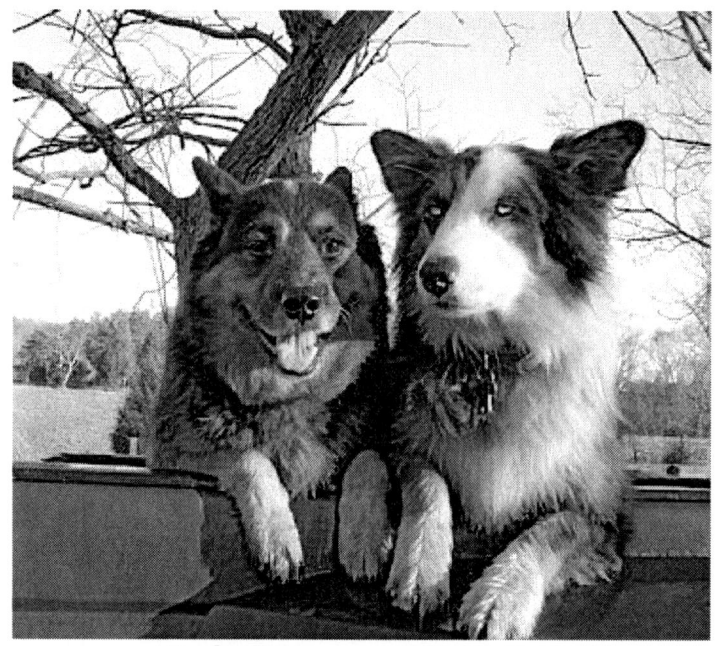

Rocky Raccoon and Spirit Dog

Rocky was never trained to herd livestock. His job was to catch and retrieve flying objects. But one day a friend who had a cattle farm explained that her new farm manager was having trouble moving two young bulls to another field. Boss Lady, whose experience with cattle is limited at best, wondered if Rocky might be able to drive the cattle into the new pasture.

A series of torrential rains had created a muddy, rocky gully by the gate and the bulls refused to go near it. The farm manager and his helper tried to get the bulls to cross the gully for a bucket of food, but the bulls just snorted and ran away.

Rocky sat patiently beside Boss Lady, assessing the situation.

"Well, let's open the gate and see what your dog can do," the farm manager said. He opened the big red gate, while his assistant opened another gate on the other side of the driveway.

Boss Lady, who had no idea what command to give Rocky, pointed to the bulls and simply said, "Rocky, bring."

Rocky sprinted under the fence and made a wide half circle around the bulls, and then he went for their hind ankles. The bulls raced forward, with Rocky like a slalom skier going from bull to bull, driving them to the gully. When one of the bulls stopped, Rocky nipped his hock, at which point Boss Lady imagined a kick that could seriously injure Rocky. But the dog was incredibly quick, and could read the bull instinctively. The bull sprang into the gully and ran up and out the gate, Rocky behind him driving him into the new pasture. Rocky turned and went back to the other bull, who was standing in the gully, mooing. Rocky darted past the bull and jumped into the gully and snapped at the bull's hind legs. This bull kicked out, but Rocky was already out of range. The dog dived in again and this time the bull leaped and galloped out through the gate and across the driveway into the pasture.

"That's some dog" the farm manager said, "we've been trying to move these bulls for two days, and your dog did it in ten minutes."

Rocky was quite pleased with himself. He trotted back to Boss Lady. He was muddy from the gully and he smelled a bit like a bovine. She gave him a big pat and a good scratch behind his ears. He wagged his tail and trotted off to find a stick for her to throw to him.

Bullwinkle was Rocky's half-brother. He was a year old and a speckled blue color, with ears that flopped rather than pricked up. He was long-coated like Rocky and had spent his life in a horse stall. The farrier who bred Bullwinkle needed to find him a home, and who better to rescue the un-socialized dog than Boss Lady? She named him Bullwinkle because she thought it was cute to have a Rocky and a Bullwinkle after one of her favorite childhood TV shows.

Bullwinkle, who was known simply as Bully Dog, fit right into the motley crew of dogs at the farm. Whether it was from his lack of socialization, no one really knows, but Bully Dog liked to herd humans. If a human wasn't moving fast enough for Bully Dog, he would come behind them barking and nipping at their knees. Sometimes his mouth would connect with jeans or bare legs. He never actually drew blood—just wails from the human and stern admonishment, at which point he would slink off, his feelings hurt.

To direct his energy, Boss Lady started throwing the ball and Frisbee. Just like Rocky, Bully Dog thought this was the best job in the world. Problem was...Rocky. He didn't think much of having a competitor in the ball-throwing, Frisbee-catching games, and he would outrun, out-jump, and out-maneuver Bully Dog, growling and barking the entire time.

So she initiated turns: Rocky in a stay while she threw the ball for Bully Dog, then Bully in a stay while she threw the ball for Rocky. Bully Dog only slightly respected the stay request. He usually interpreted it as *stay for five seconds, then go get a drink of water or lie down under a tree and wait for my turn."*

Try as she might, Boss Lady could not reach Bully Dog on a heart-to-heart level. He held himself apart; he was happy to have food, a dog bed, space to run around with the other dogs, a good game of fetch, but he clearly did not consider her "his human." She felt that the dog considered her his own concierge, and nothing more.

It can be quite complicated when a dog and human relationship isn't what either or both expected. There were times that Boss Lady thought she had failed Bully Dog, and yet there was no winning him. And that might have been their relationship for many years if Carrie Spotted Eagle had not moved in for the summer. Carrie was a long-time friend of Boss Lady's who had recently left a bad relationship and needed a place to land.

The first day Carrie moved in, Bully Dog took a shine to her. In fact, right from the outset, he claimed her as his. Where she went, he went. When she sat down to eat dinner, he laid down beside her. If she went out to work in the garden, he was right there with her. Never once did he try to herd her. *"You need me,"* he said.

At first Boss Lady was surprised at Bully Dog's rapt affection for her friend. The tug of jealousy was there; why was he drawn to Carrie and not her? Insecurity raised its head. She felt she had somehow failed this dog, or maybe that she was somehow not worthy. Grappling with insecurity meant either pushing it aside and ignoring it or taking a long look at herself, and peeling the layers. Or, as Boss Lady says, "opening up the old steamer trunks."

Possessiveness is a powerful force. It can come via material things, in the desire to hang onto stuff. It can come in the form of a pet—the need to own something living—and in ownership, sometimes the needs of the pet become secondary to the possessive longing of the person. Possessiveness can create a kind of blindness to what the animal really needs.

On a summer evening, Rocky and Ravenwolf lay in the shade of the barn eaves, watching Carrie and Boss Lady in the vegetable garden. Bully Dog lay in a spot of dirt near the corn patch watching Carrie pulling weeds. Boss Lady was in the tomato patch looking for a ripe tomato. She called out to Carrie that she had found one, and her friend came over. Just as Boss Lady snaked her arm forward to pull the plump tomato from the vine, Carrie's hand touched her wrist.

"Did you ask permission from the mother plant?" Carrie said.

Boss Lady's arm recoiled from the fat tomato. "No, I completely forgot."

"Asking is our respectful way of being," Carrie said.

Boss Lady stared at the tomato plant and said softly, "Mother, may I take one of your children?"

At that moment, Bully Dog jumped over a zucchini plant and eased himself between staked rows of tomatoes so that he was now behind Boss Lady. She turned around to look at him, and from somewhere inside her she said, "Bully, do you want Carrie to be your human?"

He wagged his tail.

There was an almost immediate sense of relief for Boss Lady, as the weight of jealousy and insecurity crumbled away like bricks she didn't know she was carrying. She called to Carrie, "Bully Dog wants you to be his human."

Carrie stood up, her long salt-and-pepper hair braid flopped against her back. She smiled, and in a sing-song voice spoke Bully's name.

The dog crashed through two tomato plants and bounded into the carrot patch, barking until he reached Carrie's side. The tomato plants he had disrupted released two ripe, fat tomatoes that rolled on the ground. Boss Lady quickly whispered, "Thank you," and picked the tomatoes up.

Months later, Carrie moved to North Carolina with Bully Dog. He was with her for a decade before succumbing to complications from diabetes. In their time together he ran between Carrie and a copperhead snake, driving the snake away and managing somehow not to get bitten himself, warned off an intruder who tried to get into the house while Carrie was sleeping, and rid her garden of groundhogs and rabbits, carefully dropping their bodies on her porch.

Rocky passed away at age 16. He had little influence on Spirit Dog, who arrived when Rocky was 11 years old. None of Rocky's obedience and dedication rubbed off on the maverick Spirit. When Rocky went blind after several years of slowly losing his sight, he did not rely on Spirit but on his own seeing-eye dog named Rutrow, a rescue from a kill shelter who looked like a dog that belonged in a Disney movie. Rutrow never left Rocky's side, and when Rocky started to get weak, he would lean against the big, fluffy Rutrow who guided him around the house and yard.

Sometimes you can find Boss Lady in the orchard, tending to the graves and markers of the dogs that have passed. Each dog has a tree and a marker where the ashes are buried. Rocky and Rutrow are side by side beneath two cherry trees. Boss Lady doesn't cry anymore when she is tending their graves. But she always says "thank you" as she touches each marker.

The Reverend Mr. Schmoo

One of the members of the pack is named Buckaroo, but his engaging personality and ability to "schmooze" humans earned him the moniker Mr. Schmoo. That name is further adulterated to variations like Schmoonie, Macarooni, and Fu Manschmoo.

Mr. Schmoo is a rather unique Aussie in that he is not interested in the typical Aussie entertainments such as chasing a Frisbee/ball/stick, pond diving, or obedience work. He will occasionally, of his own accord, do a little chicken roundup, but most of the time he likes to just hang out in the shade or on an air conditioning vent, and in the winter lie outside to enjoy the brisk, cold air.

His passion in life is eating. He can suck down the contents of his food bowl in milliseconds, the canine equivalent of a Dyson vacuum cleaner. Once he's done, he goes on reconnaissance, staking out the other food bowls as each dog finishes. He is never pushy or aggressive; he stands patiently, his eyes darting from food bowl to food bowl to gauge when the next bowl will become unoccupied and available. He swoops in, tongue ready, to lick every last nano-particle of food off the stainless steel. He is better than a Brillo pad.

Mr. Schmoo is an opportunist: sneaking cat turds out of the litter box, raiding the barn stalls for ripe manure apples, snacking on the pond grasses for an extra bit of super-green food, following Thunderbear to the secret location of chicken egg nests in the barn, and standing on his hind legs to grab some cat food off the cat table while the human's back is turned.

Mr. Schmoo is always on a diet. When Peter was doing all the dog feeding, a generosity of food poured into Mr. Schmoo's bowl. Then Boss Lady came along, exchanged his adult bowl for a puppy bowl and drastically reduced his intake….or so she thought. One morning she watched Peter fill that puppy bowl to the brim. As he turned to the sink, she started scooping huge amounts of food out of it and giving it to Thunderbear and Crockett. Then Peter turned back to the food bowls and saw what she had done.

"How can you do this to him?" he said. "He's just full-bodied, like William the Fridge."

"William the Fridge?"

"William 'The Fridge' Perry, defensive lineman for the Chicago Bears," Peter replied.

"So what are you saying, he's Mr. The Fridge Schmoo?"

"No, I'm saying you have to feed him like the big dog that he is."

"He's on a diet," said Boss Lady, and crossed her arms, meaning that the topic was no longer under discussion.

Peter turned to the pack, remembering a particular character from *One Flew Over the Cuckoo's Nest,* and dubbed Boss Lady "Nurse Ratched".

From that moment on, Nurse Ratched has been in charge of feeding and what Peter calls the draconian approach to canine weight loss. It is no surprise that Peter's pockets are crammed full of treats that he sneaks to Mr. Schmoo.

For some reason that no dog in the pack can explain, Mr. Schmoo has taken to going down to the pasture's run-in sheds on Sunday mornings and barking endlessly at the horses. The horses completely ignore him, and so he barks louder. This new habit has driven Nurse Ratched crazy, which results in Peter having to go out and call Mr. Schmoo in. Of course, whether Mr. Schmoo actually pays attention to the call is a fifty-fifty shot. Banging on a stainless steel food bowl can help.

One Sunday morning, as Mr. Schmoo was barking up a storm down in the run-in shed, an exasperated Nurse Ratched said, "I don't know why he does this, and only on Sundays. It is so peculiar and *irritating*." She stressed the last word in case Peter missed her body language of clenched fists and kitchen floor pacing.

Peter was on his second cup of French-press coffee. He stroked his beard for a moment and said, "He's preaching. It's Sunday, and he's the reverend, down there preachin' the gospel." He took a sip of coffee. "Every Australian shepherd knows that horses are sinners."

Peals of laughter ricocheted off counter tops and appliances.

"The Reverend Mr. Schmoo," Nurse Ratched chortled.

"Out there preachin' fire and brimstone from the Good Book," Peter said.

From that moment on, Mr. Schmoo has been known as The Reverend Mr. Schmoo. When he is served his puppy-bowl-size meals it is called *receiving the sacraments*. If he heads down to the run-in sheds to bark at the horses it is referred to as the *Sermon on the Mount*. When he goes into the pond with the other dogs, he is *performing a baptism*. At night when the coyotes sing and the Reverend barks loudly, it is known as *preaching to the choir*.

Not long after the Reverend Mr. Schmoo was given his full title, a strange car drove up the driveway. The pack sounded the alarm. The Reverend and Thunderbear escorted the car to a spot near the walkway while Crockett and Kemosabe barked from the confines of the house. Two young men sat in the front seat. The driver's door opened slowly as Thunderbear circled the car barking his greeting/warning. The Reverend just stood by the driver's door.

The two young men slowly got out of the car.

"Nice doggy", the driver said to The Reverend.

The Reverend just stood there. He considered turning on the charm, but decided that calmly holding the space between himself and the stranger was more in line with the dignity and respect of a dog of the cloth.

From the barn, Nurse Ratched approached the vehicle and saw pamphlets in the hands of the driver. That meant either real estate agent, lost dog, or missionary work from the Jehovah's Witnesses or Church of Latter Day Saints. As she got closer to the driver, she saw a heading in bold letters on one of the pamphlets.

"Can I help you," she asked.

"Is this dog friendly?" the driver asked.

"Depends on what sins you've committed," Nurse Ratched responded, silently chuckling to herself.

The driver gave her a puzzled look.

"That dog is The Reverend," she explained. "The Reverend Mr. Schmoo."

"Well, we're from Kingdom Hall in Orange. We're here to tell you about the Good News."

Nurse Ratched moved to stand next to The Reverend. "I'm sorry," she said sweetly. "We are not interested."

"This is an important message for you," the driver continued, flipping a page of one of the pamphlets.

"All non-secular matters here at the farm are the duty of the Reverend," she explained.

"But that's a dog!" The passenger blurted out the obvious, glancing quickly at Thunderbear, who had thoroughly sniffed him and was now checking out the contents of the car. The driver cast a withering glance at the passenger. It was hard for him to tell whether the woman was just crazy and therefore in special need of his ministry, or just playing with him for her own amusement. Either way, she really did need to hear the Good News.

"I would be happy to share the Good News with you and the er, uh… Reverend," he said, holding another pamphlet near the dog's head.

"Oh, he doesn't read," she said. "He listens to the Bible on CD and he has watched the movie *The Ten Commandments* on TV."

"I can read him this very important passage about God's Kingdom," the driver responded.

She knelt down next to the Reverend, who turned to look at her and lean into her. She whispered in his ear. He licked her cheek. Slowly she stood up.

"The Reverend says he has pressing matters with several members of his congregation that require his attention. He very much appreciates you stopping by." She turned to look at the Reverend. "What?" She nodded her head. "Oh, I see," she said, as he lowered his head. "The Reverend suggests that if you seek his counsel, please bring food."

The driver thrust the pamphlets into Nurse Ratched's hands and motioned to the passenger to get in the car.

"Please read these handouts to the Reverend. He may find them very interesting. He can contact us at Kingdom Hall in Orange."

The car drove slowly down the driveway. Thunderbear followed for a few yards, then returned to Nurse Ratched. The Reverend felt the sudden urge to roll and scratch a specific itchy spot near his tail. He flopped on the dusty driveway and let his back do the rhumba.

It occurred to Nurse Ratched right then and there that the Reverend had passed on to her an important spiritual message: getting grounded was a simple matter of rolling in the dirt from time to time.

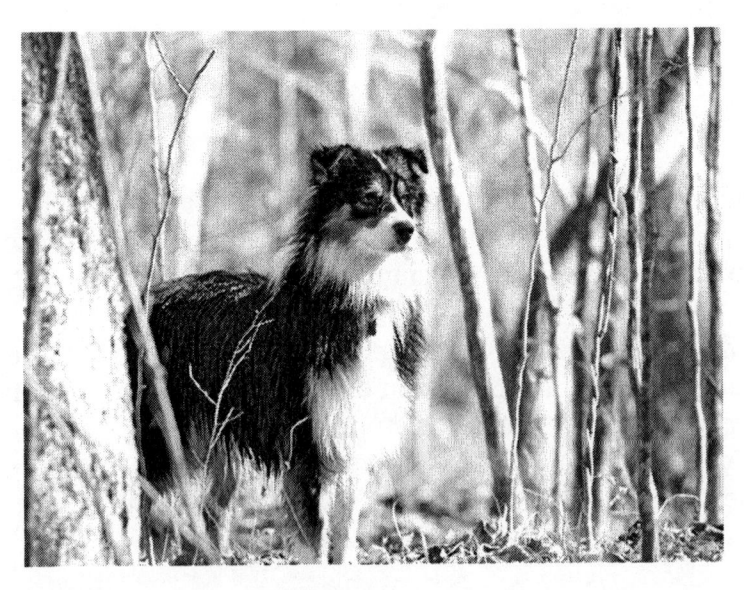

The Reverend

Part II

Nutrition and Recipes

Food, Glorious Food

It is no secret that most dogs love food. Mealtime should be an adventure for dogs, the anticipation of what will be in their food bowls. It could be cooked chicken or venison, or raw buffalo, or a prepared blend of raw organ meats, ground bones, vegetables, and fruit. It may be salmon, or chopped sardines, or eggs from the farm's chickens, either scrambled up or served whole and raw. Or, a meal could be cooked sweet potatoes mixed with beef and some cultured milk, like *kefir*.

For breakfast the dogs might get eggs and *lassi,* the fresh blended yogurt that is a traditional Ayurvedic food. For dinner it might be raw, ground rabbit with organic pumpkin puree. There could be a stew that's been slow-cooking in the crockpot all night or bone broth poured over a small portion of organic California white rice mixed with a generous serving of sautéed, or raw organic ground turkey.

Sounds like canine fine dining, doesn't it? There are actually reasons for feeding dogs this way: the long-term health of the dog, reducing the chances of dogs developing food allergies, supporting a diverse colony of microflora in the GI tract, and potentially avoiding the development of picky-eater syndrome.

Kibble

Kibble is the number one selling form of dog food. It is simple to feed, and convenient. Some brands are considerably better quality than others, although based on marketing claims it is difficult to distinguish quality kibble from what I refer to as kibble junk food.

Grain-free used to be one identifier between premium kibble and Macdonald's for dogs kibble. But now a majority of dog food kibble brands offer grain-free choices so grain-free does not in and of itself distinguish quality from junk food.

A quality, premium kibble for me means: *clean*. No ingredients labeled as *animal byproduct meal, meat byproduct meal, animal fat, chicken byproduct meal*. It cannot have *soy or vegetable oil*. It cannot have *corn or wheat gluten, corn syrup or rendered fats*. It cannot contain *propylene glycol or food dyes or preservatives such as ethoxyquin, propyl gallate, gallic acid, or propyl ester, BHA, BHT; no digest, or animal digest, or flavor, flavorings, or natural flavorings*.

The dark side of dog food

Ingredients labeled as "animal byproduct meal", "meat byproduct meal", and "animal fat" are rendered remains of dead dogs, cats, sheep, pigs, skunks, rats, raccoons, and even zoo animals. Some of these dogs and cats were euthanized, and then processed with the drugs still in their tissues, or their flea collars still attached. They are cooked at high temperatures to make soup, with chemicals added as the batch continues to boil. The meat and bones are sent to a hammer-mill press that breaks up the mass into a gritty powder, which is then called "animal byproduct meal", or "meat byproduct meal". The soup also produces tallow that is skimmed off and labeled "animal fat".

To further understand the dark side of dog food, we have to look at who is behind ingredient and labels. While the FDA is responsible for regulating pet foods, it has limited enforcement resources and is focused on human food safety. Another organization comprised of regulatory officials and major feed manufacturers known as the Association of American Feed Control Officials (AAFCO) is responsible for enforcing state laws and regulations concerning animal feeds.

AAFCO is a voluntary-membership organization whose advisors and committee members include representatives from feed manufacturers and ingredient suppliers such as Nestlé Purina, Hill's Pet Nutrition, Nutro Products, and Cargill Animal Nutrition. As Boss Lady says, "It's like having a fox in the hen house." AAFCO does not perform any analytical testing of foods, yet their regulations are adopted by most states and are the standard to which pet and livestock feed manufacturers must adhere.

The nutrient requirements were based on those established by the National Research Council Committee on Animal Nutrition in 1991. AAFCO changed the standards in 1995. One of the most remarkable changes was lowering the minimum protein content from 22 to 18 percent. Protein is clearly one of the most expensive ingredients in dog food;

by lowering the minimum protein content, dog food companies saved themselves money.

AAFCO regulations require that pet food must have a guaranteed analysis on the label and a list of ingredients presented in descending order by weight. This can be confusing to consumers particularly when it comes to protein. Rather than identifying protein sources with various parts of the food animal (muscle, heart, bone), the AAFCO regulations allow meat meal, meat digest, fat meal, bone meal and animal byproduct meal which can come from sources such as chicken beaks, pig ligaments, or intestines from diseased animals.

Remember, ingredient listings are based on weight not volume. Pet food companies can take a high-weight ingredient like corn or wheat and break it into separate parts such as bran, meal, and gluten. This allows them to move those lower-weight components farther down the ingredient list. A food can be 40 percent corn, yet the ingredient list will make it appear as though the protein source, at only 20 percent, is the main ingredient.

Understanding commercial dog food protein sources

Beef and bone meal
These are byproducts of beef parts not suitable for human consumption; considered an inexpensive, low-quality ingredient that can boost the protein percentage.

Blood meal
Pet food companies are not required to disclose the animal blood meal comes from, or what residues of medications or other substances the blood might contain. Blood meal has wide applications as a fertilizer.

Chicken byproduct meal
This can be heads, feet, bones, underdeveloped eggs, or intestines, but does not include meat. This is important, as "byproduct" in this context means any part of the animal other than meat.

Fish meal
It's impossible to know what type of fish unless specified. All fish meal not destined for human consumption must be conserved with the preservative ethoxyquin.

Poultry byproduct meal
This can be from any slaughtered fowl. Byproducts consist of parts of the animal other than meat.

Poultry meal
Not defined as slaughtered; can be obtained from dead, diseased, disabled, or dying fowl prior to slaughter.

Preservatives

BHA and BHT
Both are used to preserve fats and oils in foods. These are possible human carcinogens shown to be carcinogenic in animal experiments, possibly due to the

compounds' oxidative characteristics and metabolites. BHA/BHT are banned from human use in the EU countries and Japan, but permitted in the US.

Ethoxyquin
Originally developed by Monsanto as a stabilizer for rubber, ethoxyquin was used as a pesticide for fruit and a color preservative for spices, and later accepted for use in animal feed. The original FDA permit for use as a stabilizer in animal feed did not include pet food and was for limited use to two years. Although many pet food companies do not list ethoxyquin on their labels, it can be present in the meats and fish used in the food. A potentially toxic substance in pet food such as ethoxyquin, fed every day, year after year, creates a cumulative exposure that can affect the liver, kidneys and fat tissues. Currently the EU has banned ethoxyquin as a pesticide. In November, 2015, the European Food Safety Authority stated that it "cannot conclude on the safety of antioxidant ethoxyquin as a feed additive for any target animals, its safety for consumers or the environment" (Byrne, 2015).

Propyl gallate
Also known as gallic acid or propyl ester, this chemical is used as a fat stabilizer in dog foods. Studies on rats have linked propyl gallate to cancer, kidney and liver problems. Some evidence exists that it may have estrogenic activity (ter Veld, 2006). Gallates are not permitted in infant or children's food in the UK.

Flavor enhancers

These are ingredients that increase palatability. They are often sprayed on kibble to ensure your dog will like the smell and taste. Some enhancers include sugar and sorbitol. Among the popular flavor enhancers are animal and poultry fat. Restaurant grease has become an important component of feed-grade animal fat. Companies that specialize in blending or rendering pick up the used grease and mix different types of fat together, then stabilize them with antioxidants such as BHA and BHT to retard further spoilage; the blended grease and fat are then sold to pet food companies. Because dogs are attracted to the smell of the fats—just as humans are to the smell of bacon or a fast food hamburger—they will eat food that would normally have them turning up their noses.

Animal digest
A cooked-down broth made from unspecified parts of dead animals. Could be goats, pigs, horses, rats, roadkill, animals euthanized in shelters, mixed with the grease from restaurants.

Propylene glycol
Often used as a flavor enhancer in pet food and treats because of its sweet taste. It is banned for use by the FDA for cat food but can still be used for dog food. It is approved as a human food additive. Propylene glycol is a moistening agent and is chemically derived from ethylene glycol, which we know better as antifreeze.

Flavorings

Food products are flavored to boost sales by creating tastes that appeal to dogs, and by making the taste short-lived so that the dog wants more. Flavorings can cover up the rather vile and unpleasant taste of highly processed animal remnants. These compounds are commonly used in processed foods and would be called "fragrance" when used in cleaning products, perfumes, and cosmetics. In fact, the same companies that create fragrances also are the largest flavoring companies in the world. According to the FDA, the terms "natural flavorings" and "natural flavors" mean:

> ...*the essential oil, oleoresin, essence of extractive, protein hydrolysate, distillate, or any product of roasting, heating, or enzymolysis, which contains the flavoring constituents derived from a spice, fruit, or fruit juice, vegetable or vegetable juice, edible yeast, herb, bark bud, root, leaf or similar plant material, meat, seafood, poultry, eggs, dairy products, or fermentation products thereof* (USFDA, 2017).

Keep in mind, the description of natural flavorings or flavors does not require that 100 percent of the flavoring be from plant or animal sources. Solvents, emulsifiers, flavor modifiers and preservatives often make up 80 to 90 percent of the flavor mixture. The emulsifiers, solvents and preservatives in flavor mixtures are called "incidental additives"—meaning the manufacturer does not have to disclose their presence on food labels.

Hydrolyzed proteins and MSG

On the darker side of flavoring additives are the *hydrolyzed proteins*. These can be in the form of *hydrolyzed yeast, hydrolyzed soy,* and *hydrolyzed chicken*. The process of hydrolyzation begins with boiling the food or yeast in hydrochloric acid, then neutralizing the solution with sodium hydroxide. This process breaks the food into amino acids. This chemical breakdown of protein results in the formation of free *glutamate*, which joins with free sodium to form *monosodium glutamate (MSG)*. This does not have to be disclosed on the label.

Natural flavors often contain MSG, or free glutamate. Hydrolyzed proteins can be hidden in crops; a crop yield-enhancing product called AuxiGro containing hydrolyzed protein and MSG is sprayed on broccoli, tomatoes, potatoes, celery, cucumbers, green peppers, strawberries and watermelon. There is no way to know if the vegetables in commercial dog food have been sprayed with AuxiGro.

Hydrolyzed proteins are now being promoted by some pet food companies as being allergen-free due to the processing, which breaks the complex proteins into simpler amino acids. The theory is that dogs with food allergies aren't allergic to amino acids, even from a food source they are allergic to. The question becomes: is hydrolyzed protein a better choice than simply removing the food protein that the dog is allergic to and using a different protein?

In any case, hydrolyzed proteins are a low-nutrient food byproduct that ultimately doesn't address the real food requirement of dogs: animal protein from muscle meat.

Avoiding MSG

MSG is a flavor enhancer that works by tricking the brain into thinking that the food tastes good. It works by over-stimulating the brain—what we call an *excitotoxin*—causing an overproduction of dopamine. MSG alters the brain's ability to respond to the signal of *leptin,* a hormone that crosses the blood-brain barrier and binds to receptors in the appetite center in the brain, regulating the system that tells the dog how much to eat. Leptin stimulates the sympathetic nervous system, which in turn stimulates fatty tissue to burn energy.

Fundamentally, by reducing the brain's ability to respond to leptin, MSG added to food means the dog will eat more, continue to feel hungry, and not feel satiated. Fifty percent of dogs in the US are overweight, and conjecture among many holistic veterinarians is that hidden MSG in dog foods may be a big contributor.

To avoid exposing your dog to MSG, check the labels on supplements and dog foods to make sure they don't contain MSG or any of these other ingredients:

    hydrolyzed protein
    protein isolate
    texturized protein
    natural flavors (like chicken flavor)
    autolyzed yeast
    hydrolyzed yeast
    yeast extracts
    soy extracts or soy concentrate
    sodium caseinate

calcium caseinate
monopotassium glutamate
glutamate or glutamic acid
disodium inosinate or disodium guanylate

In addition, the following ingredients often either contain MSG or create MSG in processing:

maltodextrin
carrageenan
protease
citric acid
corn starch
gelatin
pectin

If a dog food or dog supplement lists "natural flavors" as an ingredient on the label, call the company and ask them to tell you exactly what ingredients make up those natural flavors. If the company admits to any hydrolyzed proteins, then you will know those proteins form MSG (Dyck, 2015).

Chow Time: What Do I Feed My Dog?

Omnivore*: from the Latin* omni *and* vorare, *meaning "to devour everything"*

Omnivores include black bears, grizzly bears, badgers, chickens, hedgehogs, pigs, possums, skunks, turtles, humans, chimpanzees, orangutans, and gorillas. Some fish like piranhas and catfish are also omnivorous.

Although they are the descendants of wolves, modern dogs are omnivores too. Our domesticated canines are, as one researcher put it, "one of the greatest opportunists on the planet."

Some people feed commercial dog food, others feed a raw diet, some feed home-cooked meals, and some feed a combination of commercial with cooked and/or raw. **No matter what canine diet is being fed, the fundamental nutritional components are the same: protein, fat, carbohydrates, fiber, vitamins, minerals, and water.**

Protein

Dogs require 22 amino acids. They are able to synthesize, through the liver, 12 of these amino acids; the other ten must be obtained from their diet, and are known as the *essential* amino acids: arginine, histidine, isoleucine, leucine, lysine, methionine, phenylalanine, threonine, tryptophan, and valine. These essential amino acids include the branched-chain amino acids (BCAAs), which are important for maintaining and building muscle.

Dogs active in agility, fly ball, and other canine sports have a higher protein and fat requirement than dogs with a more sedentary lifestyle. Hunting dogs, herding dogs, working dogs, sporting dogs, and sled dogs can utilize a higher protein and fat diet for their energy, endurance, and muscle requirements. Lactating mothers and puppies also need more protein.

Protein Quality

The protein percentage on a label does not equate with protein quality. The list of ingredients from a variety of commercial dog foods that provide protein sources can include items like fish meal, animal digest, corn germ meal, corn gluten meal, poultry byproduct meal, rice, chicken meal, meat meal, as well as grain protein sources like rice, barley, and oats.

Fish meal, chicken meal, poultry meal, meat meal are created through the rendering process. Depending on the process used, rendering—which is sort of like cooking a stew—can include some unsavory ingredients like flea collars, antibiotic residue or a variety of pharmaceuticals used to treat the animal before it was slaughtered or euthanized. The critical thing to remember is, *no meal product can be better than the raw material used to make it.*

Look for fish meal labeled with the type of fish used (salmon, herring, menhaden, etc). Poultry meal could be a blend of chicken and turkey, and meat meal and animal digest could be anything. When a company lists what specific animal or fish the meal is from, it is generally a higher quality protein.

Keep in mind that there are only a handful of commercial dog food producers in the US, and they own the majority of the major dog food brands. This could be one reason for the variety of companies subject to so many recalls of commercial dog food.

Fats

Fats are used by the body as an energy source, and are also necessary for the normal development and function of cells, nerves, muscles, and body tissues. Fats are made up of building blocks called essential fatty acids, including *omega-3* and *omega-6*.

Typical sources of omega-3 fatty acids in commercial dog food can include fish oils (herring and salmon), as well as flaxseed and canola oils. Typical sources of omega-6 fatty acids include pork fat, poultry fat, animal fat, safflower oils, sunflower oils, corn oils, soy oils, and vegetable oils. Grains like oats and barley also supply omega-6 fatty acids.

Animal fat, poultry fat, and the oils

Animal fat, as defined by the Association of American Feed Control Officials (AAFCO), is "obtained from the tissues of mammals and/or poultry in the commercial process of rendering." Since companies aren't required to identify their mammal fat sources, the fat could come from diseased animals, slaughterhouse waste, dead zoo animals, or even road kill. Rendered fats could also come from euthanized cats and dogs. Remember, rendered animals can be processed into meat meal, which can also be used for chicken feed which, once the chickens are rendered, can be used for fat in dog food.

Unless they are specifically labeled as organic, soy oil, vegetable oil, corn oil, and canola oils are from genetically modified organisms (GMOs). They are processed with a solvent called *hexane*, which is listed as a neurotoxin. In addition, the heat of processing destroys most of the beneficial nutrient components of the oil, including any fat-soluble antioxidants.

Flax oil, hempseed oil, and coconut oil are generally GMO-free, although a long-abandoned variety of genetically modified flax has been recently identified in several countries that imported the flax from Canada. Most flax oil is expeller-pressed, but there is still a fair amount of heat generated during the expelling process. Hempseed oil is predominately cold-pressed, maintaining its nutrient integrity. Coconut oil can be processed with hexane unless it is labeled organic, or it is verified as cold-pressed oil.

Fish oils are processed under heat, and some companies use a CO_2 extraction method that combines pressure and heat to concentrate the amount of omega-3 fatty acids. The higher-quality fish oil companies use a molecular distillation process to remove dioxins and heavy metals such as mercury. And may also use flash distillation, which uses steam rather than a vacuum to remove impurities.

Fiber

Fiber is not considered as essential a component of the canine diet as protein and fat are, but it is still a component although a small one in percentage.

There are two types of fiber: soluble and insoluble. Soluble fiber dissolves in water and forms a gel, which slows down digestion. Slower stomach emptying may have a beneficial effect on blood sugar levels and insulin sensitivity, which is particularly important for dogs suffering from diabetes. Soluble fiber sources include legumes, oats, rye, barley, some fruits, vegetables, flaxseed and nuts. Insoluble fiber does not dissolve in water, and has a stool-softening/laxative effect. Insoluble fiber sources include whole grains, beans, peas, skins of potatoes, and some fruits.

Note that meat does not contain fiber of either type; in the wild, carnivorous wolves get their fiber from the skin, hair, and intestinal contents of the animal they are eating.

The fiber sources most often found in commercial dog foods include: beet pulp, grain hulls, whole grains, flaxseed, fruit pectin, oat or wheat or rice bran, psyllium, powdered cellulose (wood pulp), and tomato pomace. Along the slippery slope of GMO ingredients, some of these fiber sources in commercial pet food include genetically modified beet pulp, rice, wheat, and other grains. Pectin is isolated from citrus and apple pomace, processed with ethanol or isopropanol, and then standardized with sugar or organic acids. Tomato pomace is the byproduct of tomato processing for juice and ketchup. Its primary component is the tomato skin, which has a higher potential for pesticide residue than the fruit itself.

As for whole-food alternatives, great fiber sources include canned pumpkin pulp (not pumpkin pie mix), steamed or cooked green beans, apple slices, and coconut meal.

Carbohydrates

If we think about the evolution of the wolf into the dog—the "wolf-dog"—we have to consider that this animal was becoming domesticated, living with or close by to humans, stealing food scraps or being fed with leftovers by the humans. Our hunter-gatherer ancestors would have eaten primarily meat, perhaps with some roots and herbs. With the advent of farming, deer would later take advantage of gardens and cornfields, but not during the time of our hunter-gatherer ancestors. Grain carbohydrates were obtained indirectly, from the digestive tracts of prey animals. However, even if the wolf-dog actually hunted down a sick, old, or young deer, the amount of grain in the intestinal tract of the deer would be minimum. Deer are browsers; they eat clover and other broadleaf plants, wildflowers, tree nuts, bushes, and bark.

As humans became more agrarian and cultivated more grains, domesticated dogs had access to stale breads and leftover porridge. Dogs living in the Far East had access to fermented soy in the form of tofu, miso, and tempeh. Over the centuries, oats, barley, quinoa, and rye have remained *relatively* unchanged, but other seeds have not. Corn, wheat, rice, and soy have been altered significantly through radical hybridization (wheat) and genetic modification (corn, rice, soy).

No carbohydrate requirements for dogs have been established by the National Research Council (NRC), and more and more companies are providing grain-free dog food. Some nutritionists and veterinarians favor grain-free, while others do not. In any case, grain-free does not mean carbohydrate free! Vegetables and fruits contain carbohydrates.

Points to consider regarding grains in commercial dog foods:

- Commercial dog foods that contain the most commonly used refined grains—wheat, corn, rice, and soy—are contributors to the decimation of soil quality via monoculture farming practices and GMO seeds. The high pesticide/herbicide/chemical fertilizer use further impacts the ecology of the soil and groundwater.

- High-carbohydrate dog foods may be less expensive in the short term than grain-free dog foods, but those carbohydrate calories add up over time. Carbohydrate information is not required on canine labels, but there is a simple way to calculate what percentage of the dog food is carbohydrates: Start with 100% and then subtract what is on the label; if the protein is 25%, the fat 15%, the fiber 4%, the moisture 8%, and the ash 3%, then the carbohydrate content is simply whatever is left. In this example, it is 45% (which is considered high...20% to 40% is considered moderate).

- Refined grains are over-processed, which destroys many of their beneficial nutrients. Also, there is evidence that excessive amounts of refined grains can contribute to obesity and diabetes.

- Minimally processed grains such as oats and barley are found most often in premium and organic dog food. Because ingredients must be listed by weight, not volume, it can be difficult for the consumer to know what percentage of grains, by volume, is in the food. The total carbohydrate amount can be calculated, but not what percentage comes specifically from grains.

- Potatoes are added to some grain-free feeds. Dogs who are overweight would benefit from avoiding white potatoes due to their high glycemic index. Sweet potatoes are a better alternative, but are still a source of carbohydrates.

Vitamins and Minerals

Vitamins and minerals are critical for the proper functioning of the body, and are involved in maintaining multiple systems including skeletal, circulatory, tissues, organs, enzymes, and the building of proteins from amino acids.

Vitamin and mineral sources

Because of the nutrient-stripping methods used in processing, commercial dog foods are fortified with vitamins and minerals in order to ensure that essential nutrient content requirements have been met. The vitamins added to most commercial dog foods and supplements are either synthetic or are byproducts of the petrochemical and coal tar industries. Because they are not from food, they are called *fractionated* or *isolated* ingredients.

Unless vitamin A is stated to come from fish oil, it is from petroleum esters. The B vitamins are taken from coal tar residue. Vitamin E, commonly sourced from palm, is extracted with hexane—a neurotoxin. Much of the rain forest of Indonesia has been destroyed by the spread of palm plantations for vitamin E production, displacing the Sumatran tiger, the Sumatran elephant, the orangutan and others. Vitamin C is made from corn or wheat and then purified through biotechnical processing into ascorbic acid. China sells the most ascorbic acid in the world.

Of all the minerals, calcium is required in the greatest amounts. Bones, egg shells, dairy products, legumes, kale, spinach, and blue-green algae are excellent food sources of calcium.

The recommended ratio of calcium to phosphorus is 1.2 to 1. Meat, chicken, eggs, and fish protein are high in phosphorus but low in calcium, with the exception of sardines, which are closer to a 1:1 ratio, but still higher in phosphorus. Other common protein ingredients like soy, turkey, duck, and lamb are also higher in phosphorus than calcium, as are cereal grains. Because of the discrepancies, balancing these high phosphorus foods with extra calcium is critical.

Mineral forms

Minerals found in commercial dog foods and supplements are most commonly present in the *inorganic* forms—carbonates and oxides—and in the *chelate* ("key-late") forms such as proteinates and amino acid chelates. These inorganic forms have low bioavailability; the body must find an organic compound to attach to the inorganic mineral before using it. This is known as *chelation*.

Plants, when they sprout, naturally bind minerals to free amino acids. The resulting amino acid-chelated minerals have a bioavailability of approximately 60%, while the inorganic forms are between 8% and 10%.

The most bioavailable forms of minerals come from food, and from amino acid chelates.

Compounds similar to amino acid chelates can be made in the laboratory, where inorganic minerals are mixed with proteins to create "proteinates." These proteinates can be labeled as chelates, but aren't true amino acid chelates because they aren't bonded to amino acids.

Ascorbates (minerals attached to ascorbic acid) are also a form of chelate. The challenge with ascorbates is understanding the GMO connection: if the ascorbic acid is made from corn, it is going to be GMO. Of course since there is no required labeling of GMOs , it is up to the consumer to contact the feed company and find out the source of the ascorbic acid.

Dog Food Diets

There are many different diets for dogs: raw, paleo, ancestral, home-cooked, vegetarian, regular canned food, regular kibble, freeze-dried raw food, dehydrated whole food, dehydrated raw food, frozen raw food...

Some owners prefer a combination diet: raw food and home-cooked, sometimes dehydrated raw with added kibble. Premium kibble can be used as a base on which to add raw, cooked or dehydrated food. For those that don't want to go all raw, the combination diet provides dogs with various sources of important proteins, fat, fiber, vegetables, and nutrients. Also, I know many other horse owners who take their dogs with them to shows and other venues. When you are spending days on the road, it makes feeding the 100% raw diet or 100% cooked diet a little more difficult, although not impossible.

Dogs with food sensitivities may do better sticking to a smaller number of proteins, but many dogs do well on a diet of rotated proteins.

Free-choice feeding

I am not a fan of free-choice feeding (the practice of making food available to your dog at all times). Owners often choose it for convenience. But if we are to feed our dog as the inner wolf he or she is, no wolf would have free-choice feeding. With the number of overweight dogs currently in the US, free feeding can only exacerbate weight issues.

Overweight dogs

Increasing exercise is important for overweight canines and humans alike. In terms of diet, dogs that are overweight need to stay below the recommended fat requirement and calorie intake. Increasing fiber will help the overweight dog feel more satisfied. Be careful with treats, as many of those dog cookies contain pro-inflammatory factors like molasses, or a high percentage of fat. Be mindful of dog food kibble that contains over 40% carbohydrates, even if it's labeled as a low-fat food.

Performance dogs

Hunting dogs, agility dogs, herding dogs, sled dogs, fly-ball dogs and Frisbee dogs require energy, and the best source of energy for these dogs is fat. Grain foods (carbohydrate energy) can create excess lactic acid in muscles and increase inflammation. Performance dogs have a higher protein requirement for tissue repair and hormone production. Higher-protein diets should be between 30% and 40% protein.

Performance dogs also have a higher antioxidant need because of oxidative stress. Antioxidant foods include: blueberries, apples, carrots, sunflower seeds (dehulled, raw, unsalted), hempseed oil, fish oil, spirulina, and microalgae (containing astaxanthin).

Adding supplements

Pet food companies maintain that their complete feeds have everything a dog needs. However, their nutritional additives are not from food, and the added minerals may only be "proteinates", not amino acid-chelated, resulting in lower bioavailability and absorption.

Adding a whole-food multivitamin/mineral will supply the necessary nutrients within the matrix of the whole food itself, thus assuring better bioavailability and absorption.

Dogs fed home-cooked food, or on a raw or paleo diet, need to supplement with a multivitamin/mineral—preferably one not derived from petrochemicals and coal tar—that provides vitamins and amino acid-chelated minerals or plant-sourced minerals.

Combination diet

If you choose to use a commercial dry dog food as a base, make sure it is premium, meaning the protein sources are identified as beef, bison, fowl, fish, and/or lamb, and are not labeled with the generic terms "beef meal", "fish meal", etc. Be sure to check the carbohydrate and fat percentages as well. There is an excellent website at *www.dogfoodadvisor.com* that rates and provides information on all commercial dog foods, along with a regularly updated list of pet food recalls. I highly recommend it.

Remember that when you add raw or cooked food to dry dog food, you must reduce the amount of kibble to adjust for the added ingredients and calories.

It's also important to add water to dry dog food, as fresh meat is loaded with moisture. If your dog was eating freshly caught game, he would be dining on a combination of blood, tissue, and organs, none of which are dry.

Companies that sell kibble claim it might clean teeth better but the facts are that 70% of dogs will get dental disease, according to Dr. Brooke Niemiec of the American Veterinary Dental College (Scott, 2017). Remember, many commercial kibble brands contain high amounts of carbohydrates and sugars. Of course some breeds are predisposed to dental disease such as toy breeds and short-nosed breeds so it becomes even more important to consider raw or combination diet.

> **The Crockpot Method**
>
> Put your protein (beef, fish, chicken, etc.) in a crockpot with some peas or lentils, or chopped green beans, some carrots, add water and cook on low, all day or overnight. Some protein sources won't require cooking as long. If you choose a tilapia fish, for example, you will only need it in the crockpot for an hour or so. Whichever meat or fish you use, the cooking water ends up making a great broth!

Adding raw food

You can add some raw bison or antibiotic-free, grass-fed ground beef either to the cooked food, or as an alternative to the cooked food. You can add a free-range, antibiotic-free egg (raw) once or twice per week. You can do a 50-50 blend of raw and cooked.

One of my favorite raw food meals for dogs is sardines with the bones packed in either olive oil or spring water. Put the sardines in a food processor along with some carrots, kale, celery, blueberries, and pumpkin meal. Mix well, and feed.

See Appendix C for further raw food recipe recommendations.

Adding fats

Fish oil is an excellent source of fat and the omega-3 fatty acids DHA and EPA. Krill oil is another fish oil source, but make sure to check that the krill has not been harvested from the oceans, which is damaging to marine ecosystems.

There can be issues with fish oil because of potential heavy metals (arsenic, lead, mercury, cadmium) in the fish oil. This is due to the toxicity of our oceans. It is critical to check with the company before you buy to make sure they will provide you with a copy of the COA (certificate of analysis) showing the levels of contaminants in their oil.

You can alternate fat sources, with flax oil, camelina oil, hempseed oil or coconut oil. Remember, our dogs are *ominvores*, capable of eating a variety of protein, fiber, carbohydrate, and fat sources.

See Appendix C for recommendations on good fat sources for dogs.

How We Got to Kibble

When dog owners think of feeding dogs in the "old days", they might imagine that canines filled their bellies with meat. In actuality, up until the advent of commercial dog food, dogs ate what the humans ate. In Europe, until the middle of the 19th century, dogs were commonly fed bread or biscuit soaked with milk or water; meat was a luxury for many people. Of course, the dogs that lived on farms had the opportunity to hunt game or steal some meat offal from a hunter's kill, lick up leftover grains from the horses' feed buckets, steal some eggs from the chicken house, and get the leftovers from human meals. The dogs that lived with royalty or lords got bones and meat scraps from the table.

The beginnings of commercial dog food

It wasn't until 1860 that commercial dog food emerged. The first of these companies was Spratt's, founded by an American in London, and specializing in dog biscuits made from grains, beetroot and vegetables. Later, the company transitioned to products with added *meat fibrine*, which was the dried, unsalted, gelatinous parts of prairie beef (known today as bison). Spratt's supplied the biscuits for the dogs serving the US army during the First World War.

Other products such as "Medicated Dog Bread" advertised themselves as "free from cheapening ingredients such as talc powder and mill sweepings". Companies like Spratt's created convenience dog food, which ultimately became kibble (Thurston, 1996).

In the latter half of the nineteenth century, dogs as pets were regarded as luxury items, and feeding pet dogs became focused on ways to "civilize" the canine race. It was acceptable that country dogs have a carnivore diet, but it was thought that meat could overexcite pedigreed lapdogs; it was believed that feeding meat would inflame their "primitive, primal passions". The feeding of prepackaged dog biscuits like Spratt's became associated with being Modern.

The advice on feeding dogs offered by the 1887 fourth edition of *The Dog in Health and Disease* by John Henry Walsh (aka "Stonehenge") might surprise many owners of today. Grains like *"Indian meal, oats, red wheat"* were boiled for 30 to 45 minutes and added as part of a broth "made from sheep's head and thickened milk". Animal food, according to Walsh:

> *...should be carefully selected to avoid infectious diseases, and the flesh of those creatures which have been loaded with drugs should also be avoided. Horseflesh, if death has been caused by accident, is as good as anything...but [animals] which have been drugged for lingering diseases and those which are much emaciated are likely to do more harm than good.* (Walsh, 1887)

Meats that were part of the canine diet in the 1800s were boiled. Only large bones were fed raw. Vegetables were recommended for dogs "to prevent their becoming overheated and getting skin eruptions". Suggested vegetables included green cabbage, turnip tops, nettle tops, carrots, and potatoes that were boiled and mixed with the broth. In *The New Book of the Dog*, written by Robert Leighton and published in 1906, the author recommends:

> *Wholesome flesh, either cooked or raw, should be the dog's stable food. It is necessary to be certain where the flesh comes from before it is distributed in the kennels and it ought always to be promptly and well boiled....wholesome butcher meat is without question the proper food. Oatmeal, porridge, rice, barley, linseed meal ought only to be regarded as occasional additions to the meat diet. Well boiled vegetables, such as cabbage, turnip tops, and nettle tops are good mixed with the meat; potatoes are questionable.* (Leighton, 1906)

Between 1890 and 1945, commercial pet foods grew as humans became more possessive of their leisure time, opting to not "slave over a hot stove" for their dogs. Oftentimes, these pet food companies utilized raw materials no one else wanted: mostly inedible meats and grains.

In the 1960s, as the dog food market grew and became more and more lucrative, American industrial giants like Quaker Oats, Ralston Purina, Armour, Swift, and several tobacco companies diversified into pet food. In order to boost sales of their commercial kibble, these companies began marketing their dog food by putting a derogatory twist on table scraps, warning of the dangers of feeding them to dogs.

By 1975, there were more than 1,500 makers of dog food, compared to 200 companies forty years earlier. In the 1980s, pet food companies declared that, according to their research, dogs actually needed whole grains and not just meat. By the 1990s, dog food companies began campaigning on the notion that *canine nutrition is a science, and best left to qualified experts*—meaning the dog food companies themselves, of course.

Horse meat for dog food

Following World War I, canned horse meat was introduced into the US under the Ken-L Ration brand name as a means to dispose of deceased horses. This brand became so popular that the company had to begin to breed horses so they could meet demand. It is estimated that, by the 1930s, 50,000 horses a year were slaughtered just to support Ken-L Ration's canned dog food production. Wild horses were also rounded up and slaughtered for canned dog food.

The arrival of kibble

In the 1950s, the first dry kibble pet foods were produced by Ralston Purina using a process called extrusion—the same process they had been using to make their Chex cereals, now applied to dog food.

By boiling meat, fat, and grain and then extruding it into the forms and sizes we know as kibble, they were able to use vast quantities of agricultural scraps from grain mills along with scraps from slaughterhouses and processing plants, including diseased meats, unusable animal parts, and meat byproducts.

The extrusion process

The extrusion process (still used today to make boxed cereals, kibble, and some snacks) is a violent one, and alters the structure of proteins. The grains and ingredients are exposed to high heat and pressure that creates chemical and physical alterations in the ingredients. This process destroys nutrients, fatty acids, enzymes, and some amino acids. When pet food ingredients are exposed to high heat and moisture during extrusion, the starch in the mixture is forced to gelatinize, or melt.

This binds the kibble and expands the product after it travels through the die of the extruder machine. The higher the starch content, the lower the density and weight of the final product. Typically, kibble dog foods contain as much as 40-60% starch. Once the kibble has dried, it is sprayed with a mixture of fats, flavors and synthetic vitamins to make the product appetizing and provide some of the nutrition that was cooked out during the manufacturing process.

Today pet food companies still use the extrusion process to make kibble. It is convenient, shelf-stable, and can be less expensive than raw or freeze-dried. Some of the industry's current innovators (such as the brands Acana and Orijen) avoid cooking at high temperatures to retain nutrient density.

Co-packers

Many dog food brands do not have their own production facilities so they outsource the manufacturing of their products. Here are some of the brands produced, listed by manufacturer, courtesy of TruthAboutPetFood.com (Thixton, 2013).

Ainsworth Pet Nutrition
Blue Buffalo
Rachel Ray

Berwind Corp. / WellPet
Holistic Select
Wellness

CJ Foods
Blue Buffalo
Castor Pollux dry (recently purchased by Merrick Pet food; it is not known if they will move manufacturing to Merrick facilities).
Drs. Foster & Smith
Nature's Variety (dry)
Rotations
Timberwolf

Diamond Pet Foods
4health
Apex

Canidae (recently purchased their own manufacturing plant)
Diamond
Diamond Naturals
Kirkland
Natural Balance dry
Nature's Domain
Premium Edge
Professional
Solid Gold
Taste of the Wild
Wellness (one variety)

Mars Petcare
Cesar (canned)
Nutro
Ol' Roy (dry)
Pedigree
Royal Canin

Nestlé
Purina
Pet Promise
Chef Michael

Proctor & Gamble
California Naturals
Eukanuba
Evo
Iams
Innova
Karma

Consolidation and megamergers

Big food companies are jumping in on the pet food bandwagon, buying pet food companies for a chance to gain a percentage of the more than $22 billion in yearly pet food sales.

In 2014, Mars, Inc.—the candy company—bought Iams and Eukanuba for $2.9 billion. J.M. Smucker (the jam company that also owns Folgers coffee, Jif peanut butter, Pillsbury, and Crisco) paid $5.8 billion in 2015 to buy Big Heart Pet Brands, maker of Kibbles 'n Bits, 9Lives, Meow Mix, Natural Balance, Gravy Train, Nature's Recipe, Canine Carry Outs, and Milo's Kitchen. Big Heart is America's biggest seller of pet snacks, including Milk-Bones, Gravy Bones, Pup-Peroni, and Snausages

According to market researcher Euromonitor International, 93% of the mid-priced dog and cat food sold in North America goes to only three companies: Big Heart, Mars, and Nestlé.

The choice of kibble

Kibble provides convenience, and one cannot underestimate the role of convenience in the food industry and in American homes.

A dog's kibble diet can be improved upon by adding table scraps (no cooked bones), some kefir or lassi, plain yogurt, some organic pumpkin meal, organic sweet potato puree, a whole organic egg, a home-cooked egg, a little hempseed oil or camelina oil or flax oil, frozen green beans, sardines, low fat cottage cheese, coconut oil, or a home-cooked breast of chicken to provide your dog with variety and less processed food.

Dog Food Allergies

Dog food allergies are on the rise; in fact, allergic reactions to food are now the third most common cause for visits to the veterinarian's office.

Remember: there's a difference between food allergy and food intolerance.

A food *allergy* is an immune response to a particular food ingredient. Symptoms of food allergy include skin rash, hives, itching, ear infections, hot spots, paw biting, obsessive licking, and sometimes nausea or vomiting. A food *intolerance* is a digestive problem, where a dog's digestive system is unable to digest a specific ingredient. Symptoms of food intolerance include gas, nausea, bloating, vomiting, and diarrhea.

Common triggers of *dog food allergies* include beef, chicken, fish, wheat, dairy, lamb, fish, corn, soy, yeast, rice, and potatoes. Common triggers of *food intolerance* include emulsifiers, flavor enhancers, dyes, preservatives, hormones in the meat used for pet food, and low quality sources of protein such as hooves, feathers, and beaks (which can be labeled as "hydrolyzed poultry byproducts" or "feather meal").

Why are dog food allergies on the rise? How do they develop?

There is a growing consensus that feeding the same diet (especially the same protein source) over a period of years contributes to dog food allergies. If you feed your dog chicken year after year, there's a good chance the dog will develop an allergy to it. Some holistic veterinarians also point to the increased use of biologically inappropriate ingredients in pet foods, including preservatives, additives, and poor-quality ingredients.

The GI tract plays a critical role in keeping out allergens and allowing nutrients to be absorbed. A healthy GI tract will break down food into amino acids, fats, and other nutrients, but if partially digested food gets into the bloodstream, the immune system can mount an attack because it views this as a foreign invader.

Going raw

Raw food is fundamentally easier to digest for dogs, because raw food contains the living enzymes that help break down protein, fats, and other nutrients. Additives, preservatives, extra carbohydrates, and the hard kibble itself can put stress on the GI tract. Raw food decreases stress on the GI tract and the body system at large, especially the immune system, thereby reducing inflammation. With so many options now available for prepared raw food for dogs, feeding raw is more convenient than ever for the time-pressed humans.

Adding marrow bones from cows or buffalo two or three times per week is important on a raw diet. Marrow bones, chicken or turkey necks provide minerals such as calcium and phosphorus, plus collagen, and they are wonderful for breaking down tartar on the teeth.

Home cooking

Home-cooked meals from a crockpot are convenient because you can make dog food while you sleep, or while you're at work. And, because you are in charge of the source of the proteins and other ingredients, you can provide a healthier meal than kibble. Using a crockpot and combining a protein such as beef, fish or chicken with some vegetables like carrots and peas is good alternative to kibble. If you use chicken, never feed the bones after cooking; they can splinter in the dog's throat or GI tract.

In terms of other supportive foods for home cooking, you can add kefir, yogurt, organic pumpkin meal, pieces of apple, whole blueberries, and sweet potatoes to your meals. Unless you have a performance dog that needs the calories, add only one additional fat source at a time: chia seeds, coconut oil, salmon oil, hempseed oil, or camelina oil.

Mix it up! Variety is important for canines. Eating the same meal day after day can create picky-eater issues and food allergies, or food intolerances. If your dog has no allergies or intolerances, offer a variety chosen from among venison, beef, wild boar, elk, salmon, trout, sardines, duck, goose, turkey, chicken, eggs, and bison. If your dog develops food intolerances or food allergies, eliminate one protein at a time to identify what protein or proteins are causing the problem.

Both raw diets and home-cooked diets need the support of a multivitamin / mineral to cover all the micro- and macronutrients.

Nutritional support for dogs with food allergies

There are specific foods that can balance the immune systems of dogs who have food allergies or intolerances:

- *Coconut oil* provides lauric acid, a potent antimicrobial and antiviral lipid converted by the body into monolaurin, which supports the immune system.

- *Bovine colostrum* provides over 80 different immune factors including transfer factors and proline-rich polypeptides (PRPs), which have the unique ability to regulate the thymus—the master gland of the immune system. Bovine colostrum provides several different immunoglobulins including IgG and IgA. With over 70 different growth factors, it also supports normal cell growth for tissue repair. (For much more information, see the "Bovine Colostrum for Canines" chapter.)

- *Reishi mushroom* is an immune system modulator that regulates the immune system and provides liver support.

- *Chicken egg yolk* (raw, organic) provides transfer factors like those in colostrum that can increase the effectiveness of the immune system.

- *Antioxidant foods and supplements* include blueberries, strawberries, apples, carrots, broccoli, spirulina, astaxanthin, pumpkin meal, sweet potatoes, whole organic eggs (raw, with shell), rosemary, and kelp.

Feeding the Overweight Dog

I noticed that Kemosabe was getting to be rather wide in the mid-section. But he was still active, running, pond-diving, and getting plenty of exercise on the farm. At first I concluded that it was because I neutered him at nine months, rather than waiting until he was two years old. I also looked at my own expanding waistline and thought, well, perhaps it's the aging process. But when I took him for his wellness check-up with my veterinarian, the scale didn't lie: he was over 80 pounds.

"Some of it is his hair," I said to my vet.

She was not moved.

We pulled blood to make sure it wasn't a thyroid issue, but everything was normal.

"You have to get the weight off of him," she said, and recommended a Royal Canin dog food for overweight dogs, which I naturally and politely refused.

Most of the time Peter feeds the dogs. I set up the supplements but he does the twice-a-day feedings. So I began to hover around the food bowls at feeding time. After a few days, I realized that Peter feeds dogs like a Jewish mother: plenty of food is a sign of love. Well, we needed to have a little less food love for Kemosabe.

So I took over. I cut the volume of his raw or cooked meals to one cup per feeding, and added kelp: one teaspoon once per day. I tried to reduce his treats to frozen beans and chopped carrots which came highly recommended and which he promptly spit out, much to my chagrin.

I chose proteins low in fat: chicken breasts without skin that I cooked in the crock pot; lean, raw buffalo; lean, cooked grass-fed beef; low-fat cottage cheese; cooked venison from a local hunter. I would still feed him commercially prepared raw food meal and added fiber foods such as organic pumpkin meal that I mixed with a little chopped kale or chopped zucchini, and some tiny slices of apple. He got hemp oil, flax oil or coconut oil because dogs need fat for energy. But rather than feed him one teaspoon of oil I gave him one-half teaspoon. I still fed him marrow bones once or twice per week, which is essential, in my mind, for dogs on raw or home-cooked meals.

The weight started to come off. When I took him to an orthopedic specialist for his elbow dysplasia, he was weighed, and had lost five pounds…in two weeks.

After four months, he was down to 58 pounds, which he has maintained even though he now gets a wider variety of foods and fats. I have increased his portion size based on his activity of the day. If we are going for a big walk in the woods and to the pond he will get more food in the morning. But I reduce the amount of food he gets in the evening because he is not burning many calories as he sleeps.

I have kept him on the kelp, which I think was a tremendous help in reducing his weight and now maintaining it. He does get treats.

See Appendix C for kelp and treat recommendations for the overweight dog.

Tips for feeding overweight dogs

- Portion control is critical, as is the quality of the food. No matter how premium the kibble is, it is not as nourishing as home-cooked or raw with ingredients you choose like you were feeding your own family.

- Kelp provides important minerals and nutrients and helps speed up metabolism by supporting the thyroid.

- If you are making a crockpot meal, make sure to skim any fat off the broth before serving.

- Frozen green beans and chopped carrots may be a good treat substitute for your dog. In Kemosabe's case, he dropped those treats on the floor and looked at me and said, "you expect me to eat this?"

- Adding fiber helps the dog feel more full without adding more fat. Avoid grains and high-carbohydrate filler foods such as potato and pea fiber.

- Bone broth is a fantastic super-food support for the gut, liver, and the joints. It makes a great supplement to a raw or home-cooked program, or as the base for a meal. I fed Kemosabe bone broth two to three meals a week during his weight loss program to provide liver support and GI tract support. It also provided a little more volume in his food bowl, so that he didn't inhale his smaller portion in two nanoseconds. (For more information on bone broth, see the "Bone Broth" chapter.)

- The amount of fat you feed daily should be cut in half for a dog who needs to lose weight. Healthy fats can be fed in small amounts. Unrefined coconut oil, cold-pressed flaxseed oil, cold-pressed camelina oil, cold-pressed hemp oil are ideal—not the inflammation-causing fats such as vegetable oil, corn oil, soy oil, or animal rendering fats, which are highly processed.

- For Kemosabe's weight loss program, I did continue feeding sardines (chopped in the food processor) but gave only one tablespoon instead of two. I also chose sardines packed in water, not olive oil.

- Choose low-fat cottage cheese and low-fat plain yogurt.

- Exercise is key to weight loss, but it becomes a challenge if your dog has joint/arthritis issues. While Kemosabe was on his weight loss program, we were in Florida for the winter and I had a very good massage therapist work on him once a week to help loosen the fascia and increase circulation.

Feeding for Healthy Skin and Coat

Nutrition is the foundation of healthy skin and coat. But what does *good* nutrition mean? It means real food, minimally processed, including a variety of proteins: beef, chicken, duck, turkey, fish, buffalo, venison, wild boar, rabbit, elk, plus fats and essential fatty acids.

A small percentage of vegetables and fruits is required as well, but dogs won't have healthy skin and beautiful coats without two critical food nutrients: protein and fat.

Protein

Proteins are made from amino acids, the building blocks of skin, hair, tissue, and muscle. A dog's hair contains 65% protein, so the sources of protein we feed are incredibly important. The sulfur-containing amino acids (cysteine, cystine, methionine) are essential for hair to grow well. Eggs, poultry, beef, dairy, and fish provide these sulfur-containing amino acids, as do legumes and some nuts and grains.

A dry coat or patches of hair loss can signal a need either for more protein or a higher quality protein. Dogs with long hair may need more protein than short-haired dogs.

Fats and essential fatty acids

Fats can fuel muscle energy, improve memory and learning, and are crucial for cell membrane health, brain health, and eye health. Essential fatty acids are fats that the body cannot produce on its own, and must get from the diet. The five essential fatty acids are *alpha-linolenic acid (omega-3)* and *linoleic acid (omega-6), arachidonic acid (AA), eicosapentaenoic acid (EPA),* and *docosahexaenoic acid (DHA).*

Deficiency in omega-3 fatty acids can lead to brain and eye issues, while deficiency in omega-6 fatty acids can lead to problems with coat and skin. Arachidonic acid is a brain fat, and too little of it can produce a dog that has difficulty learning. Eicosapentaenoic acid plays an important anti-inflammatory role in the body, and is linked to alleviating depression. Like the other omega-3s, docosahexaenoic acid is essential for eye and brain function; a deficiency can affect eyesight and mental acuity.

> **Food sources for the essential fatty acids**
>
> - Omega-3: flax, chia, hempseed, camelina oil, hempseed oil
>
> - Omega-6: sunflower, safflower, hempseed, camelina oil, hempseed oil.
>
> - AA: part of the Omega-6 family, found in meat, poultry, eggs.
>
> EPA and DHA: both part of the Omega-3 family, found in salmon, herring, sardines.
>
> As you can see, camelina oil and hempseed oil both provide the omega-3s and omega-6s. But camelina is higher in omega-3 than omega-6, while hemp oil is higher in omega-6 than omega-3. Soy and corn are also omega-6 sources, but are not recommended unless they are organic and cold pressed.

Before you think to yourself, *how am I ever going to remember all this*, here's an easy guide to feeding essential fatty acids:

Protein from ruminants
If you feed beef, bison, lamb, boar, elk, or venison, then you need to add additional omega-3s and omega-6s. In particular, lean beef, bison, and venison don't provide enough fats. Good fat sources would include hempseed oil, hempseeds, sardines, and salmon oil.

Protein from poultry
If you feed chicken, duck, eggs, or turkey, you need to add more omega-3 fatty acids (flaxseeds, chia, camelina oil, sardines, salmon oil).

Sardines and salmon oil
Sardines provide both DHA and EPA fatty acids, plus minerals in a whole food matrix. Sardines provide both omega-3 and omega-6 fatty acids. While the amounts of DHA fatty acids and EPA fatty acids in salmon oil are less than in sardines, salmon oil can be an alternative to sardines. For some dogs, salmon oil can upset the digestive tract, so introduce it slowly.

Note that fish oil supplements have some issues such as rancidity, oxidation, and processing. There are some environmental issues with krill oil; harvesting wild krill from the oceans can deprive mammals such as whales of an important food source.

Coconut oil
This type of fat provides medium-chain fatty acids (MCFAs), particularly *lauric acid, caprylic acid, capric acid, myristic acid,* and *palmitic acid*. The MCFAs provide antibacterial, antiviral, and antifungal properties. Medium-chain triglycerides like coconut oil fuel muscle and organ energy, making this a great choice for athletic dogs as well as overweight dogs, because the fat will be used for energy. Coconut oil improves digestion, and supports a healthy shiny coat. The kind of coconut oil you use is important; virgin or extra-virgin is best. Avoid refined coconut oil.

When you feed kibble...

Commercial dog foods primarily provide omega-6 fatty acids from vegetable oils and animal fats. Adding a source of additional omega-3s (flax, chia, camelina oil, sardines or salmon oil) is necessary. A study published in 1994 evaluated and proposed the optimal ratio of omega-3s to omega-6s in a range from 1:5 up to 1:10. A more recent study published in 2013, however, highlighted that the ratio was not as influential as the type and amount of omega-3 fatty acids. In other words, you don't need to drench the kibble (or cooked or raw food) in flax oil. A small amount of quality, cold pressed oil, or a small serving of flax or chia seeds goes a long way.

Rotation is key

One of the best ways to support healthy skin and coat is to rotate proteins and rotate fats. Variety is important to your dog's GI tract—specifically the microbiome of the GI tract.

Sample rotation feed plan for healthy skin and coat (for dogs weighing 40-65 pounds)

- *Day 1, AM feeding*: chicken/duck/turkey patties with 1 teaspoon camelina oil or 1-2 teaspoons chia seeds

- *Day 1, PM feeding*: beef/pumpkin patties with 1-2 teaspoons camelina oil or salmon oil

- *Day 2, AM feeding*: raw bison (grass fed) mixed with 1 whole organic egg with shell, 1 tablespoon organic sweet potato puree, 1-2 whole sardines with skin, and 1 teaspoon coconut oil

- *Day 2, PM feeding*: venison slow cooked in crock pot with peas and chopped carrots, 1-2 teaspoons hempseed oil (and 1 teaspoon coconut oil, since venison is a low-fat protein)

The shampoo conundrum

Over-bathing dogs can cause their hair to dry out. Many shampoos have a few ingredients known to be skin supportive, such as oatmeal and shea butter, but also come with a host of chemicals and sudsing agents that are just another assault on the skin.

Avoid these shampoo ingredients:

- *Cocamide DEA* or *cocamide MEA*, which can be hormone and thyroid disruptors.
- Preservative ingredients such as *diazolidinyl urea, imidazolidinyl urea* or *quaternium-15*, which break down and release *formaldehyde*; banned in Europe as carcinogenic; also cause allergic reactions and contact dermatitis.
- *Isopropyl alcohol*, which dries the skin, upsets moisture balance, and is a skin irritant

- *Methylchloroisothiazolinone (MCI)*, a preservative and known carcinogen banned in Canada and Japan; also linked to an epidemic of skin allergies
- *Mineral oil*, a petroleum product that can prevent the skin from breathing, or from eliminating toxins
- *Methylparaben* and other *parabens*, which are endocrine disruptors
- *Polyethylene glycol (PEG)*, used in the paint and coatings industry; can enter the bloodstream through broken skin and affect the central nervous system
- *Polysorbates* created with ethylene oxide, which is a carcinogen; *polysorbate 20* has 20 parts ethylene oxide, and *polysorbate 80* has 80 parts ethylene oxide; material safety data sheet indicates "may cause cancer based on animal test data"
- *Propylene glycol*, a preservative that can easily penetrate skin and weaken protein and cellular structure; can cause skin irritations, dermatitis, and hives
- *Sodium laureth sulfate, sodium lauryl sulfate, ammonium laureth sulfate,* suspected to be an environmental toxin; a known skin irritant with small molecules able to cross cell membranes; can be corrosive to fats and proteins

Getting dirty

When dogs roll in the grass, the dirt, mud, manure, and dead animal carcasses, they expose their largest organ, the skin, to bacteria, soil organisms, and soil fungi. The incredible diversity of microorganisms in the skin and GI tract of dogs is critical to their health. Let your dog get dirty! Hose the dog off with water and be careful not to use antibacterial soap with *triclosan*. We know on the human side that the use of antibacterial soaps with triclosan has been shown to disrupt the gut microbiome, and a plentiful, diverse gut microbiome is critical to a healthy immune system.

Canine skin problems on the rise, and what we can do about it

Skin problems such as atopic dermatitis are steadily rising in frequency, and although there can be a genetic component to skin allergies passed down from mother or father to puppies, genetics are not the whole story. What we feed to support the immune system, what lifestyle our dogs have, and the extent of our dogs' exposure to chemicals via pet shampoos, environmental toxins, and household cleaners all play an important role in either stressing the immune system, or reducing stress on the immune system.

Allergies are a major cause of skin problems, specifically dermatitis, which fundamentally means inflammation of the skin. Sometimes this can be a flea bite, hot spots, parasite infestation, hypersensitivity, food sensitivities, even allergies to grasses, molds, and environmental allergens.

Remember: for dogs, having healthy skin and a healthy coat begins in the gut! Providing nutritional support is important:

- Change the diet, feeding one protein at a time to gauge whether there is a food-protein sensitivity.

- Feed the microbiome of the GI tract with active live probiotics such as kefir or unsweetened yogurt. Probiotic supplements of at least 1 billion CFU per serving and that contain multiple strains of active microorganisms will help recolonize the GI tract.

- If your dog is on a kibble food, make sure it is grain-free and provides a single protein source.

- Increase omega-3s in the dog's diet and add coconut oil for immune support.

- Supplementation with bovine colostrum can be beneficial to regulate the thymus.

- Even if you can't feed a 100% raw diet, add some raw food to your kibble or cooked food to provide live enzymes for the gut.

- Manage stress with herbs such as holy basil and ashwaganda.

- Help reduce inflammation with turmeric and boswellia.

- Don't forget the super-green foods like kale and spirulina for their antioxidant and anti-inflammatory properties.

See Appendix C for specific recommendations for foods and other products mentioned in this chapter.

Bone Broth

Bone broth is one of the super-foods for dogs. It is wonderful for a convalescing dog, makes a perfect addition to raw or cooked meals, gives kibble more nutritive value, and lends support for healthy joints and GI tract. Bone broth provides the important amino acid *glycine*, which the liver uses for detoxification—a process that can be limited if there isn't enough glycine. In fact, glycine deficiency may reduce the liver's ability to synthesize bile.

Bone broth also provides *glycosaminoglycans* that support and maintain collagen, along with a compound known as *glucosamine*, which is found in many canine and human joint formulas, and is needed to form glycosaminoglycan and *hyaluronic acid*.

Bone broth can also help support leaky gut syndrome due to the high content of gelatin, which helps plug the tight junctions in the gut that can get larger due to stress, bacterial imbalance, and poor diet. Leaky gut exposes the body to undigested food and toxins that the body then starts to attack. This begins a syndrome of food sensitivities, allergies, and immune stress.

Bone broth is easy to make:

1. Cover the bottom of a crockpot with bones. If you have a lot of dogs, you will want to fill the crockpot

with bones. Turkey wings and legs and marrow bones are good choices...I use all three together. Some people use chicken feet with additional wings and legs added. Joints of the type found in wings and legs are important sources of *glucosamine sulfate*.

2. Add enough water to cover the bones by two inches, add 2-3 tablespoons of apple cider vinegar (raw with the mother). If you are cooking a large pot of bones, add 3-4 tablespoons of raw apple cider vinegar.

3. Cook in the crockpot on the high setting for 1 hour, reduce to low for 23 hours.

4. When the broth is finished, strain the bones, removing any meat by hand. *Do not feed the bones to the dogs!* If you are worried about the fat, just skim it off the top before straining.

5. You can add vegetables to the bone broth after it has finished cooking and before it cools. Chopped kale, green beans, celery, and carrots are good choices. Once the broth is cool, you can refrigerate or serve.

Refrigeration will give the broth a jelly-like consistency. You can freeze bone broth, or keep it in the fridge for several days. You can also use ice cube trays to keep the bone broth frozen for when you need it. These little individual broth-sicles can be fed when it's hot outside and you want to provide a nutritious, cooling treat.

Feeding for the Kidneys

Kidneys process waste products and water, which then go the bladder and are released as urine. These organs are important regulators of sodium, phosphorus and potassium, releasing them back to the body to maintain homeostasis.

Kidney disease is becoming more prevalent in dogs. One of the early signs of kidney disease is the intake of more water by the dog. When the kidneys aren't functioning properly, more water is needed to flush out the toxins. This increase in water intake can lead to dehydration, lethargy, loss of weight, appetite, even vomiting or diarrhea.

A routine blood test by the veterinarian can detect kidney disease by measuring levels of *blood urea nitrogen* (BUN) and *creatinine*. Urea is a waste product produced in protein metabolism and eliminated by the kidneys. Creatinine is a breakdown/waste product of *creatine phosphate* in muscle. The kidneys filter and remove creatinine, so testing for this substance estimates how well the filtration process is working. Elevated BUN and creatinine values are due to increased levels of waste products that indicate possible kidney disease.

What to feed: high-protein versus low-protein

Commonly, vets recommend a low-protein diet because protein is high in phosphorus. Studies on rats have shown that restricting dietary protein prevents progressive kidney failure. However, dogs are omnivores while rats are primarily herbivores. A double-blind study compared actual kidney function, creatinine levels, body condition and survival time of dogs fed a low-protein diet (16%) versus those fed a moderate-protein diet (22.5%)—both diets with restricted phosphorus content. They found no significant difference in kidney function, creatinine levels or survival time between the two groups. Body condition scores were greater for the moderate protein group because they maintained muscle mass. The determining factor in survival time was the level of kidney dysfunction at the time of diagnosis, not the diet (Tudor, 2013).

An interesting part of this study is that the low-protein diet used was still higher in protein than common commercial diets formulated for kidney disease. This indicates that muscle wasting would be even more pronounced in diets with lower than 16% protein.

Of additional importance, this study shows the relevance of phosphorus, and how controlling intake of this particular mineral is more critical than controlling protein.

Phosphorus

Because reducing phosphorus is critical in the management of kidney disease, reducing or eliminating high-phosphorus foods is important. Remember, we do not want to eliminate all phosphorus in the diet, because it is an essential nutrient.

- High-phosphorus foods include organ meats, bones, sardines and egg yolks. Stay away from quinoa, millet, brown rice, and oatmeal, as they are high in phosphorus as well.

- Moderate-phosphorus foods include ground beef, chicken breast, chicken thighs, ground pork, green tripe, whole milk kefir, eggs without the yolks, cauliflower, pumpkin, cabbage, and sweet potatoes.

- Low-phosphorus foods include tapioca, sticky rice, apples, blueberries, cucumbers, and coconut oil.

Calcium and phosphorus

Maintaining the optimal 2:1 calcium-to-phosphorus ratio is important. Calcium can bind phosphorus, but you would not want to feed more calcium if your dog already has elevated levels of the mineral (hypercalcemia). Egg shells, either ground or broken, are excellent whole-food sources of calcium. Do not use bone meal or dicalcium phosphate because the phosphate is too high.

Sample meals for feeding the kidneys

These recipes are for a 50-pound dog, and can be adjusted accordingly.

I. 6 oz. ground beef (grass fed, 20% fat), cooked
   4 oz. sticky rice
   2 oz. winter or summer squash, cooked
   1 egg white
   1 egg shell, crushed
   1 tablespoon blueberries
   (can be divided into two 1-cup meals)

II. 6 oz. chicken (white or dark meat), cooked
    4 oz. organic sweet potatoes, cooked and pureed
    1 oz. chopped kale, raw
    1 oz. whole milk, yogurt, or kefir
    1-2 apple slices
    1 egg shell, crushed
    ½ teaspoon coconut oil

III. 6 oz. green tripe, raw
     3 oz. organic pumpkin puree
     2 oz. cauliflower, cooked
     1 oz. raw cucumber, chopped
     1 oz. tapioca (prepared with water)
     1 egg shell, crushed

Supplements

It is important to make sure your dog is getting all the micro- and macronutrients, so adding a good whole-food multivitamin/mineral is important. You will also need to add an active probiotic and an omega-3 and omega-6 oil (see Appendix C for recommendations).

What to avoid when feeding for the kidneys

- Avoid feeding dry food, which can increase dehydration in dogs with kidney issues.

- Avoid kibble because the additives and petroleum-sourced vitamins can increase the toxic load.
- Avoid canned food because of carrageenan and flavorings. Research published by the Jesse Brown VA Medical Center in Chicago showed that carrageenan induced an inflammatory response in human and mouse epithelial cells (Bhattacharyya, 2014).

- If you must feed kibble, add some home-cooked chicken or beef and low-phosphorus veggies. Make sure the kibble is moist to support good hydration.

Feeding for the Liver

The liver is an organ that is responsible for metabolizing fats, cleaning and filtering the blood, and synthesizing proteins. The liver has the amazing ability to regenerate and heal itself, but environmental toxins, toxic substances, bacterial or viral diseases, cancer, pancreatitis, and even medications can all put stress on the liver.

Liver disease is not uncommon in dogs. Because the liver cleans the blood, toxins such as herbicides and pesticides that the dog is exposed to, or long term use of certain pharmaceuticals can put the liver at risk. It is important to get a diagnosis of liver disease from a veterinarian who can run the appropriate tests and biopsy if necessary.

Particular dog breeds such as Great Danes, Dalmatians, and Labrador retrievers can be more susceptible to liver problems due to their genetic inability to excrete copper.

The standard, low-protein approach

Often, it is recommended to feed dogs with liver disease a low-protein diet. Yet protein is needed by the liver for regeneration and repair. In fact, the issue isn't protein—it's *ammonia*.

Certain protein sources are low in ammonia, while others are high. It is important to supply quality protein with sources that are low-ammonia, such as **eggs, low-fat yogurt, low-fat cottage cheese, poultry without the skin,** and **fish**. Beef is the highest ammonia producer, and should not be fed. This is especially important for dogs with chronic liver disease.

Reducing fat

Lowering the percentage of fat in raw or home-cooked meals is essential in helping the liver heal. Feeding a low-quality fat such as vegetable oil or animal rendering fat could put more strain on the liver. Remove fat from any poultry protein you are feeding (such as the skin on chicken) and choose low-fat dairy foods. Remove the yolk from eggs, especially for dogs that have chronic or late-stage liver disease. You don't want to completely eliminate fat, as it is still an essential nutritional component.

Adding fiber

Some commercial dog food companies with specialty formulas for liver disease use more carbohydrates than protein. It is best to focus on complex carbohydrates that provide sources of fiber, both soluble and insoluble.

Good choices for soluble fiber include **oatmeal, cooked lentils, cucumbers, celery, apples,** and **blueberries**. Good choices for insoluble fiber include **brown rice, couscous, broccoli, zucchini, pumpkin meal,** and **cabbage**.

Sample meals for feeding the liver

These recipes are for a 50-pound dog, and can be adjusted accordingly.

I. ¾ cup cooked salmon or cod
  ½ cup cooked oatmeal
  ¾ cup low-fat cottage cheese
  ½ cup cooked broccoli or cauliflower
    Mix well and serve

II. ¾ cup cooked chicken without skin
  ½ cup organic sweet potato, canned or fresh, then baked or boiled
  1 egg (without yolk for dogs with chronic liver disease); can be cooked; if fed raw must be organic, free-range
  1 egg shell, crushed
  ¼ teaspoon flax oil
  ¼ cup diced apples or apples mixed with blueberries
    Mix well and serve

III. ¾ cup cooked ground turkey
  ½ cup cooked brown rice or couscous
  ½ cup chopped mixed celery, carrots, and cucumbers; can be raw
  ½ cup low-fat yogurt
  1 egg (without yolk for dogs with chronic liver disease); can be cooked; if fed raw must be organic, free-range
  1 egg shell, crushed
    Mix well and serve

With advanced liver disease, it is best to feed four small meals a day rather than two large meals. In this case, the above large-meal recipes can each be split into two small meals.

Supplements

The water-soluble vitamins such as vitamin C and the vitamin B complex are important support for the liver. The fat-soluble vitamins such as vitamin E and vitamin A also need to be supplemented. A good whole-food multivitamin/mineral will provide your dog with these important nutrients. (See Appendix C for recommendations.)

Remember, the source of a nutrient is important, especially for dogs with health issues. Adding vitamin A that is petroleum-sourced, or B vitamins made from coal tar just puts more stress on the GI tract.

Milk thistle

Milk thistle is an important herb for the liver. It helps repair as well as prevent damage to this essential organ. It is important to know that milk thistle is a medicine; it is an herb that is only used for a specific amount of time. A dog without liver issues does not need milk thistle, and should not be given the herb as a preventative.

Extracts of milk thistle are preferred over the dried herb because of the concentration of the active substance *silymarin*, a potent antioxidant. Silymarin has demonstrated membrane-stabilizing action, reduction of the inflammatory reaction, and inhibition of fibrogenesis in the liver (Féher, 2012).

Extracts of milk thistle contain 70-80% silymarin. Check with your veterinarian regarding dosage. Generally, the daily recommendation is ¼ teaspoon per 20 pounds of weight. It is best to divide the dosage evenly into smaller portions and give two or three times per day. Most tinctures are alcohol-based, so diluting the dosage with water can reduce the unpleasant taste.

Monitoring weight

If your dog starts gaining weight on the liver-supportive food diet, just reduce the amount of food. If your dog is losing weight, increase the amount. You want to be able to feel your dog's ribs as a gauge of a healthy weight. You do not want to see the ribs.

Remember, food quality is important for healing. Feed your dog what he or she needs for the liver to heal and repair.

Feeding for the Pancreas

The pancreas regulates sugar and digestion; this organ produces insulin that controls blood glucose, and is responsible for making digestive enzymes that are necessary for the metabolizing of protein, carbohydrates, and fats.

There are two diseases involving the pancreas, not including pancreatic cancer: pancreatitis and diabetes.

Pancreatitis

In fundamental terms, this is inflammation of the pancreas. If the enzymes produced by the pancreas are activated prematurely, they will digest the pancreas itself. In severe cases, the enzymes are forced out of the pancreas into the abdominal cavity where they can start breaking down fat and proteins in other organs such as the liver and kidney.

If your dog is showing symptoms such as loss of appetite, diarrhea, vomiting, and/or arching of the back, it is very important to get to a veterinarian immediately for a precise diagnosis. As you can see, the symptoms mimic other disorders such as gastritis (inflammation of the stomach lining).

Causes of pancreatitis

- Some breeds are genetically predisposed: miniature schnauzer, cocker spaniel, Yorkshire terrier, and miniature poodle are among the breeds that are more susceptible.
- Overweight dogs and dogs with Cushing's disease are at greater risk for developing pancreatitis.
- It is more common to see pancreatitis in middle-aged to older canines, as well as in females.
- Some medications may also affect the pancreas, including *prednisone,* the *tetracyclines, long-acting antacids, diuretics,* and *acetaminophen.*
- There is some evidence that exposure to organophosphates, which are commonly used as insecticides, can cause inflammation of the pancreas.
- Dogs with diabetes can be prone to pancreatitis.
- A dog can get pancreatitis from gorging on garbage or eating inappropriate foods.

Types of pancreatitis

There are two basic forms of pancreatitis: acute and chronic. Acute is limited to one incident, while chronic refers to several acute occurrences. In both cases, you will need to reduce the amount of fat in your dog's diet. Some holistic vets recommend fasting the dog for 24 to 48 hours after an occurrence, still giving them access to water so that they won't dehydrate.

Reducing fat

It is important to reduce the fat in your dog's diet with diseases of the pancreas:

- Avoid fatty foods like lamb and pork.
- Trim fat off poultry, use only white meat, feed extra-lean beef.
- Use egg whites.
- Use low-fat cottage cheese and low-fat plain yogurt.
- Beef kidney and beef liver are low-fat, but use only small amounts together with another low-fat protein source.

Foods to support recovery from pancreatitis

It is best to feed three or four small meals a day for dogs with pancreatitis. This puts less stress on the GI tract at large and the pancreas specifically. In cases of acute pancreatitis, you may only need to do this for a few weeks before gradually transitioning to a regular food plan of two meals per day. Dogs with chronic pancreatitis should be fed three or four meals per day for life.

By volume, you want to feed at least 50% protein, 25% vegetables, and 25% starch. You can vary this, of course, to 50% protein, 30% vegetables, 20% starch or other proportions as long as the protein is the highest percentage by volume. I am careful with starchy foods, and I would not feed them in a volume greater than the vegetables.

Protein sources include white meat, poultry without the skin, low-fat beef or buffalo, small amounts of organ meats (beef kidney, liver, heart), egg whites, low-fat cottage cheese, and low-fat plain yogurt.

Vegetable sources include pumpkin meal (freshly cooked or canned, preferably organic), cooked spinach, cooked broccoli, cooked cabbage, cooked zucchini, cooked summer squash, cooked kale, and cooked collard greens.

Starchy food sources include sweet potatoes without the skin, oatmeal, rice, and barley. *If your dog is diabetic, do not feed these grains. Please see the chapter "Feeding the Diabetic Dog" for more information.*

Sample meals for feeding the pancreas

These recipes are for a 50-pound dog, and can be adjusted accordingly. Each recipe should be divided into 3 or 4 servings.

I. 1 cup white chicken meat, cooked
   ½ cup low-fat cottage cheese
   ½ cup cooked sweet potato without the skin or canned organic sweet potato puree
   ¼ cup zucchini, cooked
   ¼ cup summer squash, cooked
   Mix well and serve

II. 1 cup lean beef or bison, cooked
   ½ cup low-fat yogurt
   ¼ cup kale, cooked

¼ cup cabbage, cooked
½ cup oatmeal, cooked
Mix well and serve

III. ½ cup beef heart, beef liver, or beef kidney, cooked and drained of fat
1 cup lean beef or bison, cooked
½ cup rice, cooked
¼ cup spinach, cooked
¼ cup broccoli, cooked
Mix well and serve

IV. 1.5 cups lean ground turkey, cooked
1 or 2 egg whites
½ cup barley, cooked
¼ cup organic pumpkin meal
¼ cup collard greens, cooked
1 egg shell, ground
Mix well and serve

Supplements

Digestive enzymes are very beneficial for dogs with pancreatitis, easing the workload of the pancreas. Make sure the digestive enzyme supplement contains *protease*, *lipase*, and *amylase*, which digest protein, fat, and carbohydrates, respectively.

Active probiotics are important for the balance of beneficial bacteria in the GI tract. On days you don't feed yogurt, give a multi-strain, active probiotic with at least one billion

CFUs per serving. (See Appendix C for specific supplement recommendations.)

Feeding the Diabetic Dog

As food is being broken down during digestion, carbohydrates are converted into sugars, including glucose. Glucose supplies the cells with energy. However, glucose can only enter cells if the pancreas-produced hormone *insulin* is present. While humans can get Type 1 or Type 2 diabetes, the form of diabetes dogs get is Type 1: the body cannot produce insulin. This disease is commonly known as *diabetes mellitus*. Without insulin, the cells cannot absorb glucose, which then raises blood glucose concentrations in the body.

Certain breeds have an increased risk of developing diabetes, including the Keeshond, poodle, Samoyed, dachshund, Alaskan Malamute, minature schnauzer, Chow Chow, beagle, Doberman pinscher, Labrador retriever, Hungarian Puli, golden retriever, miniature pinscher, Old English sheepdog, springer spaniel, schipperke, Finnish spitz, West Highland white terrier, and cairn terrier.

By some estimations, one in every 500 dogs will develop canine diabetes. While canine diabetes can be genetic, it can also be caused by poor diet and obesity. A diet with high carbohydrates and poor protein sources can be a contributing factor.

The treatment for canine diabetes is insulin injections, as directed by the veterinarian—generally every 12 hours.

Diet for the diabetic dog

Because the pancreas is involved, the diet needs to include quality protein and lower fat. But we also need to keep the carbohydrates low; it is better to feed low glycemic vegetables like crookneck squash, zucchini, and cabbage, and to avoid the higher glycemic foods like oats, barley, and rice.

Sample meals for feeding the diabetic dog

These recipes are for a 50-pound dog, and can be adjusted accordingly.

I. 1.5 cups low-fat ground beef or buffalo, cooked
   ¼ cup yellow squash, cooked
   ¼ cup zucchini, cooked
   ¼ cup non-fat yogurt or non-fat cottage cheese
   Mix well and divide into 2-3 feedings per day

II. 1 cup white meat chicken without skin, cooked
   ½ cup chicken livers, cooked
   ¼ cup cabbage, cooked
   ¼ cup zucchini, cooked
   1 egg white, cooked
   1 egg shell, crushed
   Mix well and divide into 2-3 feedings per day

III. 1 cup low-fat ground beef or buffalo, cooked
   ½ cup beef heart or beef liver (can be fed raw or cooked)
   ¼ cup spinach, cooked

¼ cup broccoli, cooked
¼ cup non-fat yogurt or non-fat cottage cheese
Mix well and divide into 2-3 feedings per day

IV. 1.5 cups salmon, cooked
1-2 egg whites, cooked
¼ cup kale, cooked
¼ cup yellow squash, cooked
1 egg shell, crushed
Mix well and divide into 2-3 feedings per day

Supplements

Kelp is important for the micro-mineral content, as is *spirulina*, which also provides macro-minerals, B vitamins, and beta carotene.

Camelina oil is an excellent source of fatty acids and vitamin E, and doesn't have the potential mercury toxicity of fish oil. For diabetic dogs, give: ⅛ teaspoon for dogs 10 pounds and under; ¼ teaspoon for dogs 11-25 pounds; ½ teaspoon for dogs 26-55 pounds; and 1 teaspoon for dogs over 55 pounds. Note that this is a reduced amount relative to most camelina oil servings for dogs (see Appendix C for dietary oil recommendations).

Feeding Dogs with Cancer

It is a staggering statistic that 50% of American dogs will get cancer. The causes for this disease are varied and include genetics, toxins, and environmental factors. I think processed food plays a role, in that high-heat processing of meats found in commercial dog foods provide lower-quality nutrition. There is also the question of the role of chemical preservatives and how they impact the immune system over the lifetime of the dog. Many ingredients in commercial dog food kibble can contain genetically modified organisms (GMOs), which have been exposed to increased levels of herbicides and pesticides. A dog consuming these toxins daily, for years, may be more at risk.

One of the goals of nutrition and real food is to put less stress on the GI tract specifically, and the glandular and immune systems at large. We want our dogs to live as long and as healthily as possible, so the food we choose and how this ultimately affects the body—the kidney, liver, bladder, passive and active immune systems, metabolism, GI tract, and circulation—is one of the most critical aspects of dog ownership.

The genetic component to cancer is complicated. Certain purebred dogs have higher cancer rates than others. If a mixed-breed dog has parentage with a high cancer rate, the chance of developing cancer in a mixed breed remains high.

Based on information from Tufts University Veterinary Cancer Registry, dog breeds in North America with higher than normal cancer rates include the golden retriever, German shepherd, poodle, boxer, Rottweiler, Bernese mountain dog, Shetland sheepdog, cocker spaniel, Doberman pinscher, beagle, miniature schnauzer, and shih tzu (Steinberg, 2017).

Scandinavian studies have indicated that breeds most likely to develop cancer include the Bernese mountain dog, boxer, giant schnauzer, standard poodle, Rottweiler, Irish wolfhound, cocker spaniel, Doberman pinscher, Pomeranian, Newfoundland, German shepherd, Saint Bernard, Great Dane, greyhound, and basset hound (Brønden, 2010).

According to the Tufts Registry, *lower* than normal cancer rates have been found in the miniature pinscher, papillon, Cavalier King Charles spaniel, Pekingese, Akita, Saint Bernard, Pomeranian, Great Pyrenees, bloodhound, Newfoundland, mastiff, bullmastiff, Chesapeake Bay retriever, Chihuahua, and bichon frise.

As you can see, some of the breeds found most at risk for cancer in the Scandinavian studies are among those the Tufts Registry lists as having a lower than normal risk. Why? It may be that gene pools within the same breed differ from region to region. This kind of information is crucial for dog breeders. Improving the gene pool of the Saint Bernard, for instance, may need to start with stock not in Scandinavia.

Environmental factors such as insecticides, herbicides, household cleaners, and solvents in paint may cause cancer in pets. The problem is, these chemicals are studied more for their impact on humans than on dogs and cats. Many chemical products that dogs are exposed to, such as flea-and-tick dip, have inert ingredients that are, or contain, known human carcinogens, including *benzene, toluene, xylene,* and *petroleum distillates.*

Research on dogs living around lawns treated with 2,4-D has shown that measurable amounts of the herbicide were absorbed by the dogs for several days after application. Whether this exposure increases the risk of cancer is unknown at this time. However, if you have a dog of a breed with higher than normal cancer rates, it would be advisable to keep your dog away from exposure to 2,4-D and other pesticides.

The World Health Organization's International Agency for Research on Cancer announced in 2016 that *glyphosate* (marketed heavily by Monsanto as Roundup) is "probably carcinogenic to humans" (IARC, 2016). In 2017, California became the first state to declare glyphosate a known human carcinogen.

Note that overweight animals are at an increased risk because many chemical compounds are retained in the animals' fat.

Feeding dogs with cancer

For dogs with cancer, it is important to feed supportive, real foods containing quality proteins, quality fat sources, and low carbohydrates. Fats cannot be well utilized by cancer cells for energy. However, carbohydrates can be fuel for cancer cells and should be fed minimally, in small amounts.

Avoid high-starch vegetables such as *potatoes, sweet potatoes, carrots, green peas, yams,* and all *grains*. Low-starch vegetables can be fed instead; these include *broccoli, Brussels sprouts, cabbage, cauliflower, collard greens, crookneck squash, kale, spinach,* and *zucchini*.

Whether you decide to go raw or home-cooked, remember to prepare your dog's meal with love and mindfulness. You are making medicine.

The raw food diet

If you choose to feed your dog with cancer a raw diet, remember that variety among proteins is important. You can feed ground bison and add chicken hearts and eggs. You can feed ground lamb and add whole milk cottage cheese and canned sardines with the bones (in water).

Bones are a critical component to raw feeding. You can feed chicken necks, wings, turkey necks, beef ribs, pork necks, and lamb ribs. *Do not cook these bones!* Cooked bones can splinter in the gut.

Feed small meals more often—3 or 4 times per day—rather than twice a day if your dog has been diagnosed with cancer.

The half-and-half diet

If you are hesitant to go totally raw, you can do half home-cooked with half raw.

Sample meals for feeding dogs with cancer

All recipes are for a 50-pound dog, and can be adjusted accordingly.

Half-and-half diet meals

A.M. feeding
    1 chicken thigh, cooked (remove bone)
    ⅓ cup ground bison or grass-fed beef, raw
    ¼ cup whole cottage cheese
    1 teaspoon coconut oil

Noon feeding
    1 can sardines with bones (in water)
    ½ cup salmon, cooked
    1 egg, raw (organic, local)
    1 egg shell, crushed
    ¼ cup plain yogurt
    1 turkey neck or marrow bone, raw (for dessert)

P.M. feeding

1 cup venison, bison, ground beef, or ground pork, cooked

¼ cup chicken or beef liver, beef heart, or beef kidney, raw

1 egg, cooked or raw

¼ cup plain lassi or plain kefir

¼ cup bone broth (for recipe, see the "Bone Broth" chapter)

Home-cooked diet meals

Crockpots are excellent for making home-made dog food, because you can cook on low for hours without overcooking and losing nutrient value. The two sample crockpot preparations below can be used as a base for the daily meals that follow.

I. In a crockpot, add:
- 1 pound ground bison, beef, venison, pork, or lamb
- 1 cup chopped broccoli or broccoli florets
- Enough water to cover everything

Cook on low for 3-4 hours, or high for 2 hours. If you want to cook overnight, just add more water and cook for 6-8 hours on low.

II. In a crockpot, add:
- Package of chicken thighs
- 1 cup crookneck squash or zucchini

Cook on low at least 5-6 hours, or on high for 3-4 hours

Refrigerate unused portions until you need them. When you are cooking organ meats, don't use the crockpot; just sauté in a sauce pan with butter or coconut oil.

A.M. feeding
    1 cup of the cooked bison, beef, venison, pork, or lamb
    ¼ cup of the cooked broccoli
    ¼ cup beef or chicken liver, or heart, or kidney, sautéed
    ¼ cup whole milk or plain yogurt
Add the water from the crockpot as a tasty, nutritious broth or add 2-4 tablespoons of bone broth.
Mix well and serve.

Noon feeding
    1 cooked chicken thigh with skin—*do not feed bones!*
    ½ cup chicken livers, sautéed in butter or coconut oil
    1 egg, scrambled
    ¼ cup of the cooked zucchini or squash
    ¼ cup whole milk cottage cheese
    1 egg shell, crushed
Add water from the crockpot as a tasty, nutritious broth.
Mix well and serve.

PM feeding
    1 can of sardines with bones (in water)
    2 eggs, hardboiled, soft-boiled, or scrambled
    ¼ cup kale or collard greens, sautéed
    ¼ cup whole milk plain yogurt or lassi
Mix well and serve.

Snacks for your dog

- Cheese (not processed cheese)
- Dehydrated liver squares (see Appendix C for recommendations)
- Hard-boiled eggs

Supplements

See Appendix C for specific recommendations regarding the following supplements:

- Spirulina for macro- and micro-minerals, plus phytonutrients and antioxidants

- Brewer's yeast or nutritional yeast for B vitamins and additional protein

- Medicinal mushroom complex (*reishi, shiitake, cordyceps, maitake*) for immune support
- Bovine colostrum for immune report and cellular repair

- Fish oil for the essential fatty acids; if you are concerned about contaminants with fish oil, use camelina oil, which not only supplies high amounts of omega-3s but also the antioxidant vitamin E.

Turmeric paste

Turmeric is a spice that provides many important benefits to the body: it reduces inflammation; it is a potent antioxidant; it supports the liver; and it supports good digestion in the GI tract. There is some evidence that turmeric can inhibit certain tumors' growth and may shrink existing tumors. The active ingredient in turmeric is *curcumin*, which may interact with some medications such as NSAIDs and blood thinners.

There are many recipes for golden turmeric paste that you can find on the internet, and they are essentially the same. Most call for 1½ teaspoons freshly ground black pepper. I only use ½ teaspoon, because the full amount was too much for the GI tract of one of my dogs. Black pepper is part of the paste recipe because it provides *piperine*, which helps the body absorb the curcumin.

The following recipe for "Golden Paste" was developed by Australian veterinarian Dr. Doug English (Scott, 2017). I have tweaked it to include a smaller amount of ground pepper.

    Ingredients:
        ½ cup organic turmeric powder with a high percentage of curcumin
        1 cup filtered water
        ½ teaspoon freshly ground black pepper
        ¼ cup organic coconut oil

Pour the water in a saucepan and slowly add the turmeric. Stir the mixture on low to medium heat for 7-

10 until it forms a paste. If it is too thick, just add a bit more water.

Remove from heat, add the coconut oil and black pepper and stir well. Allow to cool. Store in a glass container with a lid. Will keep for two weeks in refrigeration, or frozen for six months.

When feeding turmeric paste, start with a small amount: ¼ teaspoon several times per day. For dogs over 60 pounds, start with ½ teaspoon. Large dogs may need a tablespoon over the course of a day.

Cannabidiol oil

There is growing evidence that *cannabidiol (CBD) oil* can support dogs undergoing chemotherapy, as well as lessen the pain and discomfort of various cancers. Dog owners have reported that their dogs with cancer have needed no pain medication other than CBD oil, were less stressed, and in some cases actually lived months longer than expected.

CBD is a component of both the hemp plant and the cannabis plant. Because hemp oil is legal in the US, some companies have been selling hemp oil as a source of CBD for dogs. Yet, according to *High Times* magazine—the bible of cannabis smokers and growers for 40 years—hemp oil does not contain as high a level of CBD as cannabis. In order for hemp to produce high amounts of CBD, hemp strains with higher CBD amounts would need to be developed and cultivated.

I was introduced to hemp oil in 2000, when a Canadian company began selling their newly launched hemp oil in US health food stores, and I was consulting for a company that was handling its distribution. At that time, CBD was poorly understood, but as more states legalized medical cannabis, more information and testing was done on CBD.

BioStar introduced hemp oil to the equine market in 2007, and then brought out hemp oil for dogs in 2012. I have a great appreciation and love for hemp oil. I think it's a fantastic oil with unique benefits such as *gamma-linolenic acid* (GLA) to help reduce inflammation in the GI tract. I love how sustainable the plant is, and how many uses it has, including clothing, food, and even house-building.

If I had a dog diagnosed with cancer, however, my source for CBD would not be hemp oil; it would be cannabis oil. Which brings up a delicate subject: in states where cannabis is not legal, what is a dog owner to do?

You can make your own CBD oil or butter. A simple Google search will return loads of how-to instructions, and a special device exists that can help you make plant butters or extracts very easily (see Appendix C for a recommendation). You do run a risk, of course, when procuring the cannabis and being assured of the strain you have purchased. Some strains are high in *tetrahydrocannabinol* (THC), and would not be the best choice. Whether to use CBD oil from cannabis is a very personal decision, and in states where it is not legal, the dog owner is committing a crime.

There are small networks springing up of people who either make the CBD oil for themselves for the cancer they are fighting, or who just love making cannabis products. These small networks will provide the CBD oil at no charge, or may request a donation to a charity.

I know a woman in North Carolina whose dog was diagnosed with bone cancer. Through a friend of a friend of a friend, she got a small bottle of cannabis-derived CBD oil and started feeding it to her dog. His appetite improved, he had less discomfort, and she was able to stop his NSAIDs medication. She was so inspired that she started growing two plants in her house, making her own CBD oil, and sharing it with other friends of friends of friends. Her own dog lived six months longer than the veterinarian had predicted.

The most important part of living with a dog who has cancer is making sure our dog's quality of life is the top priority. In our human-ness, we sometimes wait too long to say farewell because we can't bear the passing.

Twenty years ago, I had a dog named Bear Dog who was diagnosed with bone cancer. I did not do the surgery for fear of the cancer actually spreading, and relied on the pharmaceutical pain medications to keep him comfortable. When I knew we were at the end—when he was no longer interested in food, the pain in his eyes was heartbreaking, and I had to increase the pain meds significantly to keep him comfortable—I invited Bear Dog's human friends over for a celebration of his life. He loved the attention and rallied to the bits of dog treats, the pats, and the Bear Dog stories, his tail wagging. The next morning the vet came.

Bear Dog was ready and he went quickly, with his head in my lap.

I regret that I didn't know about raw and home-cooked meals then. I didn't know about CBD. But his passing spurred me to learn a lot more about dog food.

Feeding Puppies

Many breeders send puppies off to their new owners when they're between eight and twelve weeks of age. Typically, the puppy has been weaned onto kibble and the breeder will recommend staying on that specific brand. Most often, puppies adopted from shelters or rescues are also on kibble, and new owners may even receive a complimentary small bag of kibble from a major dog food company. Since the puppy is going to experience many changes all at once, it is a good idea to keep the puppy on the kibble at least for a few weeks. If you want to start adding real food, you need to do it slowly.

When I bring a puppy home, I feed kibble and give the puppy time to adjust to his/her new surroundings. Some puppies adjust quickly and others take more time. My youngest dog, Crockett, was so distracted by the other dogs eating that he forgot about his own food bowl. Sometimes he would wander around and check on why the other dogs were eating so voraciously. If a cat wandered by, he'd leave his food bowl and follow the cat. Sometimes, when he would stare at his bowl of kibble, and then at the others dogs eating their home-cooked or raw meals, I got the impression he was saying, "How come I have to eat this stuff?" When I started adding some home-cooked food to his kibble, Crockett got a lot more focused on eating.

There are breeders who start their puppies off with raw food during weaning. Sometimes their purchase contracts state that the puppy continues on a raw diet after the dog goes to its new home. These breeders are very experienced with raw food for puppies and are excellent sources of information.

Feeding large and giant-breed puppies

Breeds that are 50 pounds or over are most often considered large breed, though I personally rank large breed as 60 pounds or more. Giant breeds are considered to be 100 pounds or more.

The nutritional needs of these breeds are not the same as the nutritional needs of small and medium breeds. Large and giant-breed dogs grow faster and remain puppies longer. This rapid growth can cause abnormalities such as orthopedic diseases such as elbow dysplasia, osteochondrosis (OCD), hip dysplasia, and developmental orthopedic disease (DOD).

Genetics plays a role of course, but so does overfeeding and excessive dietary calcium. It's important to remember that calcium in kibble (mostly in the form of calcium carbonate) is not the same as calcium from bones. First of all, raw bones provide other cofactors such as silica, sulfur, magnesium and phosphorus, as well as gelatin, which is a form of extracted collagen.

Very good information about feeding large and giant-breed puppies (including a calcium calculator) can be found at the website DogFoodAdvisor.com. (See Appendix C for details on this and other excellent resources for feeding large and giant-breed puppies.) The information in the remainder of this chapter will be geared to feeding medium and small-breed puppies.

Kibble with raw or home-cooked added

You can begin by adding some home-cooked food to the kibble: a little cooked chicken mixed with canned organic pumpkin, or cooked bison with organic canned squash. Sometimes I'll add some whole-milk cottage cheese, a little bit of cooked egg, or some kefir. Adding home-cooked food does require lowering the kibble amount by about one quarter. You aren't replacing the kibble, you are simply fortifying it with real food.

I may occasionally throw in a tablespoon or so of the raw food the adults are getting, as well as a tablespoon of sardines with the bones. In addition, I will *gradually* introduce the puppy to cooked beans, raw frozen beans, cooked carrots, and raw carrots, either as part of a meal or as a treat.

With my new puppy Wookie, I began immediately adding raw to the kibble and skipped the home-cooked food. I really do believe that feeding raw is the best food for canines.

It's important to read your puppy. Fat puppies are cute when they are eight weeks, but as they grow they should get leaner. I go over the puppy's body with my hands at least once a week. I want to feel the ribs, but not see them. I also feel the shoulder blades, the top line, and assess the health of the coat.

At this stage—say, from eight weeks to five or six months—I add only a multivitamin mineral supplement to the feed plan and occasionally a little salmon oil or camelina oil two or three times per week if the puppy is healthy and looks great. If the puppy is thinner than I like, or the coat is dry or lackluster, I will increase the protein and add a more fat: coconut oil, salmon oil, or camelina oil.

Raw only

If you want to start off raw, there is a legion of opinion on the internet that favors not adding raw to kibble for puppies. One theory is that a puppy should be eating all raw or all kibble. I personally don't subscribe to this belief because the ancestors of our dogs and their puppies were eating raw when they caught a rabbit and eating cooked meat when they hung around a human's camp. I wean my puppy off kibble and onto all raw, but I take my time doing it and pay attention to the puppy's appetite, feces, behavior, and speed of growth. While I believe feeding raw is the best way to feed dogs because it is the healthiest food for them, I do take time to transition.

Whether you decide to feed kibble or raw to your puppy, or a combination of both, the best recommendation is to start with one protein source such as poultry and let your puppy's GI tract adjust to that for a couple of meals before introducing a new protein.

Some puppies can adjust to new proteins quickly, others that have more sensitive GI tracts may take longer. But you do want to rotate proteins, and combine proteins to avoid picky-eater syndrome and potential food intolerances.

Just say no to dry kibble

I never feed kibble dry. If my dogs were living wild, they would take down prey and eat muscle, hair, intestines, blood. It would not be a dry meal. I always wet the puppy's kibble either with water, or some broth left over from a crockpot meal, or some diluted goats milk or kefir. Frankly, this notion that dry kibble helps clean the teeth is a myth. Dry kibble contains a lot of carbohydrates, which do not breakdown plaque and tartar. What does break down plaque and tarter are the enzymes in raw meat and bones. Some breeds are predisposed to tartar build up, particularly short-muzzled and toy breeds.

From four months on…

By the time the puppy is four months old, I have eliminated the kibble entirely and feed raw and or home-cooked food. By this time the puppy has been exposed to different foods, so increasing the volume of these foods does not upset the digestive tract. Since the puppy has already been given a diet mixed of kibble and raw or kibble and cooked I move to all raw with an occasional cooked meal. Commercial raw dog food options have just exploded on the market, and this makes feeding raw very easy. One of the benefits with commercial raw food for dogs, other than convenience, is that muscle and organ meats are usually included, as well as ground bone, fats, and veggies which provide a very balanced raw food meal. (See Appendix C for a list of some highly rated and recommended raw food brands and products for puppies.)

Supplements

As the kibble is reduced, you'll need to add a multivitamin / mineral supplement, preferably one made of whole food ingredients.

If the puppy will be traveling, I will start a probiotic the day before, such as whole milk plain yogurt or kefir. If it is going to be an overnight trip, I will use a multi-strain probiotic and not a single-strain as yogurt and kefir are. Since the micro-biome of the GI tract is comprised of literally billions and billions of microorganisms of various strains, it makes sense to provide multiple strains to maintain a balance in the GI tract, particularly when the puppy is under stress.

I will add some omega-3 oil (salmon oil, flax, or camelina oil) at ¼ teaspoon for every 20 pounds of body weight. I also rotate my omega-3 sources; sometimes it's salmon or fish, sometimes flax or camelina.

Treats

I used to be a bad treat feeder. I'm embarrassed to say that before I paid attention, I just fed treats like Milk-Bones, other grocery store dog treats, and rawhide chews. I classify these kinds of treats as pure junk food and avoid them like the plague.

Rawhide treats are dangerous because they can cause blockages and choking. And there is another dark side to rawhide treats: they are a byproduct of the leather industry, which means they have been chemically bathed, processed, and bleached. In a way, every rawhide treat provides low-dose toxins that can accumulate over time in the fat cells of the body.

I give puppies freeze-dried or dehydrated beef liver treats that are easy to break into small pieces, little bits of goat's milk cheese, slices of carrot or green beans, raw or cooked.

I do introduce raw bones at this point: turkey necks, chicken necks, chicken backs, and beef neck bones. *Never feed cooked bones to your puppy or dog!*

I make frozen coconut/peanut butter treats for the dogs, but only introduce them to puppies at around five or six months due to the fat content. It's a simple recipe: 1 cup liquefied coconut oil (organic) and 1 cup organic smooth peanut butter. I mix it well and spoon into silicone molds, which can get messy, but then I love peanut butter and coconut oil so I don't mind using my fingers to wipe up the over-fill. You can also pour the mixture into a plastic baggie and snip one corner to squeeze it more precisely into the molds. Once frozen, the treats pop out of the molds easily and you can keep them frozen in a separate container. (For the plump puppies, mix 1 cup canned organic squash meal with 1 cup canned organic pumpkin meal, pour into silicone molds, and freeze...makes a tasty lower-fat treat.)

My dogs love marrow bones, femur bones, and knucklebones. It is critical when offering these bones to match the dog with the size of the bone. Small marrow bones for an aggressive chewer would not be as wise a choice as a big beef knucklebone. The small femur ring marrow bones commonly found in grocery stores can be swallowed whole by some of the larger breed dogs, or those dogs that have strong vertical bite force. Bigger bones are better.

The marrow in marrow bones is high in fat. You can scoop out the marrow for puppies (or dogs) if you need to watch their waistlines. Replace the marrow you have scooped out with canned organic pumpkin meal or canned organic squash meal and freeze. Now you have a significantly lower fat content. You can also stuff the scooped out marrow bones with peanut butter and freeze if your puppy does not have overweight issues.

Getting trained by your puppy

It happens to most of us: the beguiling puppy we brought home turns out to be a master manipulator that we don't even suspect until the puppy is totally running the show. I used to think that puppy classes were for first time owners. Every puppy who came into my life learned basic commands and I was satisfied if "stay" lasted a couple of seconds.

Having Aussies taught me that there was a great deal about dog training I didn't know. In many ways these dogs are smarter than I am. I did not take Kemosabe to a puppy class with a professional trainer but I have now done puppy classes with the three youngest Aussies: Thunderbear, Buckaroo, and Crockett. Do I really need to go to these classes now that I've done it multiple times? Yes. And now that I have a new puppy I will go back to Puppy 101 class. First and foremost for me I get reminders of things I've forgotten from a puppy class three or four years ago. Secondly, puppy classes are great for the needed socialization of puppies under supervision. And thirdly, there is the human socialization of spending time with others who love their puppies.

There are benefits with a training system, particularly one that isn't aggressive; I personally prefer positive reinforcement training. In a wholistic training class the puppy gains socialization skills; the human gets reminders of that which she/he forgot, or learns a new way of approaching a problem; and, it's just plain fun to be with other people and their puppies, learning from their mistakes as well as their successes.

Real food and compassionate, timely training turn a happy puppy into a happy dog.

Tigger Montague

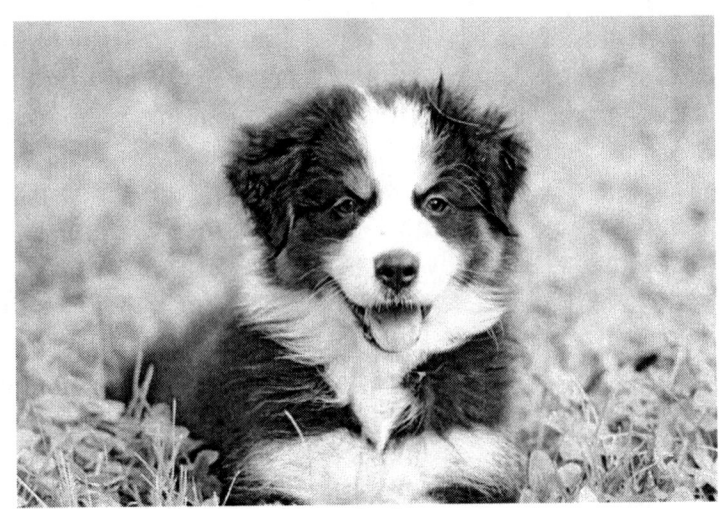

Thunderbear

Going Raw

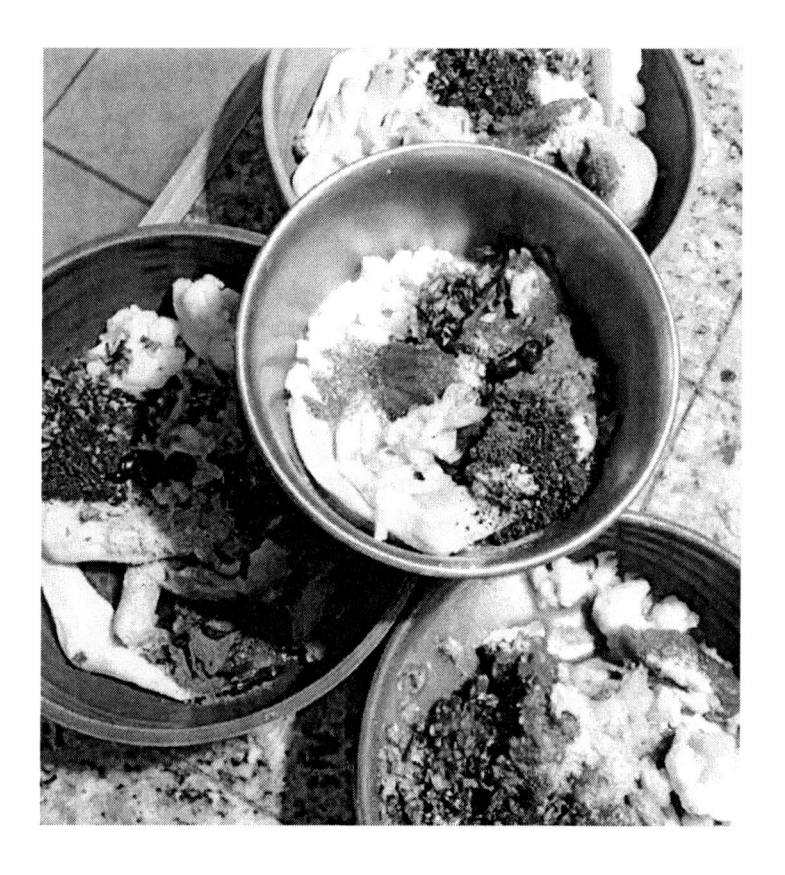

I eased into raw with my dogs, starting first by adding it to home-cooked, and then finally taking the leap and going all raw. Although I understood raw from a nutrition standpoint, and I agreed with the concept of feeding an ancestral diet, I was a little nervous. So if you're not currently feeding raw, and are tentative about it, you're not alone.

What tipped me over the edge to going all raw with my dogs was a summer evening while watching the horses graze. The horses were eating raw, unprocessed grasses: the most essential and important food for equines. Why was I not providing my dogs with the same essential-to-their-species foods?

Feeding raw at first glance seems complicated. And feeding multiple dogs raw seems overwhelming. Luckily, raw food for dogs has been made easy by the arrival of some pretty cool raw food companies who make feeding raw almost as easy as feeding kibble—and so much better for the dogs!

I do make some raw meals that don't come out of a bag (I think the dogs would stage a protest if they didn't get their sardines mixed with pumpkin meal at least once a week), and I enjoy the prep time, with the dogs gathered around asking, "Is it ready yet?"

One of the biggest differences I've seen in my dogs since going raw is their stool. There's a lot less of it to pick up. The reason for this is that their bodies are utilizing more of the food because the enzymes in the raw meats, bones, and organs help digest the food in the gut. The larger the amount of poop being excreted, the less food is actually being digested. Feeding home-cooked meals can reduce the amount of poop compared to kibble, and going raw means there will be even less, as your dog is able utilize a greater proportion of what you feed.

The brain-gut connection

Many raw food advocates say that anxiety-ridden dogs and hyperactive dogs become calmer and more settled on a raw diet. From a nutritional point of view this makes sense, as we know on the human side that highly processed meals for children can exacerbate hyperactivity and even some learning problems. The gut is the second brain.

Researchers at the Johns Hopkins Center for Neurogastroenterology are finding evidence that irritation in the GI system can result in signals sent to the central nervous system that trigger mood changes. Their work focuses on the *enteric nervous system* (ENS), which is comprised of two thin layers of more than 100 million nerve cells that line the gastrointestinal tract from esophagus to rectum—more neurons than are found in the spinal cord.

In addition to the neural network of the GI tract, there is a whole ecosystem made up of trillions of gut bacteria that communicate with these enteric nervous system cells. This is important when choosing what to feed our dogs because the more varied the diet, the greater the diversity of bacteria. We know on the human side that people who eat mostly processed foods have a less diverse community of bacteria in the gut than those who eat a variety of unprocessed foods. We also know that humans eating mostly processed foods have increased levels of a specific bacteria phylum called Firmicutes. Obesity has been linked to high Firmicutes numbers in both mice and humans.

Research has shown that the enteric nervous system uses more than 30 neurotransmitters, and that 95% of the human body's serotonin is found in the bowels. Serotonin maintains mood balance in humans and animals (Hadhazy, 2010).

Veterinarians and raw food

An increasing number of veterinarians are recognizing the health benefits of a raw diet for dogs; however, there are still many veterinarians who shy away from raw food and will happily steer a client to the various veterinary brands like Royal Canin and Science Diet. Some of the resistance from veterinarians is due to fear. It's far easier to recommend a bag of kibble than it is to provide a guide to raw food feeding. Some of the fear comes from being limited to their own vet school educations, where raw diets are simply not part of the curriculum.

The irony of this is that the original "BARF" diet—Biologically Appropriate Raw Food—was created by a veterinarian named Dr. Ian Billinghurst. In his practice, Billinghurst came to the conclusion that "the further an animal's diet departs from its evolutionary diet, the more health problems that animal is likely to develop. That is why modern grain-based pet foods, no matter how well researched, cause so many health problems." (Billinghurst, 2012)

Standing up for your dog

During the winter of 2017, I was in Wellington, Florida with two of my dogs, Kemosabe and Crockett. For two days Crockett had very loose stool, but he was normal in every other way. I added some kefir to his food and organic pumpkin meal, but by the third day he had projectile diarrhea, and Kemosabe's stool, which had been firm, was now loose.

Since my vet was in Virginia, I made an appointment with a new practice in the area and brought the dogs in. The veterinarian asked what I was feeding, I told him raw, and he said, "well that's the problem."

It wasn't the problem. As the stool sample showed, there was no *Salmonella* or *Clostridium* present. Blood work was normal. He put the dogs on antibiotics and told me to feed cooked chicken and rice. I did this for three days, and although there was no more projectile diarrhea, Crockett's stools were still not formed on the cooked chicken and rice.

I went back to the vet, who immediately accused me of still feeding raw. When I told him I was feeding *his* diet, he switched the antibiotic.

Another week went by with no improvement in Crockett. Kemosabe was better, but his stools still weren't normal. I made an appointment at another vet clinic to get a fresh take on my dogs, and had the records from the first vet sent over.
The new vet commented on how healthy my dogs looked and complimented me on the fact that they were not

overweight. He looked at their teeth and gums and commented on how healthy their mouths were, with no sign of gum disease or tartar buildup.

After checking the stool samples I had brought, he switched antibiotics once again and added a Panacur wormer, although results from the previous vet showed no high worm counts. When he asked me about feeding them, I told him they had been on raw but now were on cooked chicken and rice with a little pumpkin meal and probiotics.

"Well," he said, "I highly recommend you put them on Royal Canin for sensitive GI tracts."

What I wanted to say right then and there was, *"Are you freaking kidding me?"* What I said instead was, "I'm sorry, I will not feed processed food to my dogs."

He looked at me like I was from Mars. "Royal Canin is scientifically formulated by canine nutritionists," he said.

"I happen to be a canine nutritionist," I told him coldly. "And let me tell you there is no real food in processed pet food."

He turned on his heel and left the examining room.

After a week of the new antibiotic and the course of Panacur, both dogs had improved a bit, but their stools still weren't normal. The dogs had been on cooked chicken and rice for three weeks and I knew it wasn't good for them to be on the same food week after week, so I went back to adding some raw, and then going all raw, as before. Their stools became normal again.

Later, I discovered that the next-door neighbor had been applying various herbicides to his lawn, in addition to hiring a professional company to spray pesticides. My dogs walked by that house almost every day on short walks, and I'm pretty sure their paws came in contact with those contaminants, which then entered their systems and disrupted their GI tracts.

Finding the best veterinarian for you and your dog

It's hard to stand up to veterinarians; in our culture they are the authority figures when it comes to animal health. They know a lot more about health issues, diseases, abnormalities, and medications that we owners do. Veterinarians are an important part of maintaining health and wellness in our dogs. Yet there are times and issues involving nutrition and vaccines where we, as owners, need to speak for our dogs.

It's important to find a veterinarian that will respect your stand. The veterinarian for my dogs does not agree with feeding raw, but she also doesn't try to cram Royal Canin down my throat, or try to persuade or guilt me into feeding processed food. I also don't agree with her recommended vaccination schedule, and so we agree to disagree. She doesn't try to bully or guilt me into giving multiple vaccinations to a mature dog, and I appreciate that—just as I appreciate her skills when one of the dogs is injured, and her compassion when it's time to say goodbye to an older dog.

Take it slowly or jump right in?

There are raw food advocates who believe it's best to go straight into raw rather than gradually introducing it by mixing with kibble or home-cooked. Their belief is that the canine GI tract can become more disrupted by blending raw with other foods.

The GI tract of dogs who eat raw meat and bones is very acidic, with a pH of 2.0 or lower. This highly acidic environment helps break down raw meats and raw bones. The low pH is also highly effective in killing bacteria, particularly pathogenic bacteria like *Salmonella*, *Clostridium*, *Campylobacter* and *E. coli*. Because dogs have a short GI tract compared to humans and horses, they can digest and absorb nutrients from raw meat in a relatively rapid transit time of 8-12 hours, whereas a horse who eats plants has a transit time of 36 hours.

When we feed kibble, with all of its plant protein and carbohydrates, we reduce the acidity of the stomach, and the pH becomes more and more alkaline. The change to a higher alkalinity slows gastric digestion and transit time. It also creates an environment where unfriendly bacteria and contaminants are not destroyed as effectively.

What this means is that a dog that has been eating kibble and is given a raw bone as a treat may have trouble digesting the raw bone material because the pH in the gut is more alkaline than if the dog had already been eating raw meat.

When I decided to go all raw with my dogs, I started slowly, adding small amounts of raw meat to their home-cooked food. I transitioned them over seven days, gradually reducing the proportion of home-cooked food and adding more raw. I had no trouble with upset tummies or runny stools. They adjusted quite readily.

Remember, my transition was first from kibble to home-cooked, and then from home-cooked to raw. My home-cooked meals were predominantly meat and fat with a tiny amount of vegetables. This kind of diet is not nearly as pH-raising as kibble. But it still doesn't produce as low and acidic a pH as feeding raw (Syme, 2017).

If your dog is on kibble and you're ready to go raw, keep in mind that whether you transition over a week or so, or jump right in, there is going to be a change in the pH of the GI tract. As the GI tract adjusts to the new food, the stool may change, and the dog may get an upset stomach. This is normal. The pH will eventually adjust, though, and then you will start noticing little things such as a brighter coat, less poop, a happier dog, and ultimately a healthier dog.

Seeking the Balance

One of the marketing techniques of the pet food industry has been to convince dog owners that dogs must have a balanced diet with every meal. I once bought into that propaganda myself, trusting that by feeding high-quality kibble I was giving my dogs a balanced diet. Frankly, I didn't know what a balanced diet was, but I figured the pet food companies did.

It was while researching wolves and coyotes that it dawned on me that balance, for the wild canids, was not provided in every meal. For a wolf, having a balanced diet happens over the seasons, varying with the vegetation the prey animals are eating. Neither do we humans eat a balanced meal three times a day. Our ancestors, even our great grandmothers before the age of globalization, ate seasonally. They had gardens, and canned a lot of what they grew for the leaner wintertime when fresh vegetables were not available. They stocked up on meat in the age of freezers and refrigeration. They didn't expect to go to the grocery store every week and buy fruit from Chile and vegetables from Mexico in the middle of January.

What is a balanced diet for dogs?

The pet food companies say their highly processed blend of proteins, fats, carbohydrates, fiber, and some vitamins and minerals provide the ideal balance for a healthy dog. Yet, as any label reader knows, some of those ingredients are suspect when it comes to quality: meat byproducts not fit for human consumption, renderings of euthanized animals and denatured oils for fats. Often there is much more carbohydrate content than dogs need, and then there are those pesky additives: coal tar and petroleum-derived vitamins, along with an array of preservatives. The guaranteed analysis on a bag of kibble does not equate to quality protein, fat, carbohydrates, or fiber.

Because I follow the ancestral diet, my dogs' meals are generally 55% protein, 25-30% fat, and 15-20% carbohydrates and fiber. These percentages aren't written in stone; one meal may have more carbohydrate/fiber content and a little less fat, while another meal might have only 10% carbohydrate/fiber, 60% protein and 30% fat.

How about vitamins and minerals?

I use a multivitamin/mineral made for adding to raw and home-cooked meals. Calcium is one of the heftier requirements for dogs, so raw bones, organic eggs with the shells, kefir, lassi, raw goat's milk, blue-green algae, and kale are good food sources.

Phosphorus is an important mineral in protein synthesis and for the production of the energy molecule ATP. The ratio of calcium to phosphorus needs to be 1:1, or even as high as 2:1. Meat tends to be high in phosphorus, so adding eggs with the shell plus another source of calcium will help balance the high phosphorus content of the meat. Raw bones are an excellent source for calcium/phosphorus, providing a ratio between 1:1 and 1.2:1.

Balance in the long run

The irony is that commercial dog food kibble, for all its marketing success as "complete and balanced", has not made our dogs healthier. Genetics play a role in longevity, of course, but the rise in rates of allergies, cancer, liver disease, and kidney disease makes what we feed and how we feed it even more important.

Feed the highest quality food you can. If you have to use kibble, add real food to it, and remember that balance is an ongoing process: real food and variety give the body what it needs to be in balance.

(See Appendix C for literature and product recommendations for balanced feeding.)

Warming, Cooling, and Neutral Foods

In Ayurvedic medicine, foods are classified as warming, cooling, or neutral (balancing). Using foods according to these classifications is very helpful when dealing with health issues and seasonal temperature changes. See the example warming and cooling foods below, and make sure to notice the neutral foods that follow, because they can be combined with either cooling or warming foods for balance and variety.

Warming foods for dogs

Think of warming foods as increasing energy in the GI tract, which is beneficial for dogs that are constipated, or dogs that are older and losing weight. Warming foods support circulation—good for dogs that get cold easily, or have arthritis, or are just moving more stiffly.

Many types of foods are classified as warming, including:

- ***Protein:*** beef, chicken (especially dark meat), saltwater fish (including sardines), turkey (only dark meat)

- ***Grains:*** quinoa, rice, wheat

- ***Vegetables:*** green beans, cooked peas

- **Fruits:** cooked apples, ripe bananas, kiwis, peaches
- **Fats (oils):** salmon oil
- **Nuts/seeds:** peanuts, sesame

Cooling foods for dogs

These are the foods that lower the heat in the GI tract and the body system at large. You would feed cooling foods to dogs that overheat, get heat stress, or who have exerted themselves in hot weather. Cooling foods are helpful when dogs have diarrhea, inflammation, or are running a fever.

Cooling foods include:

- **Protein:** white chicken meat, freshwater fish, rabbit, white turkey meat, venison, egg whites.
- **Grains:** oat bran, pasta, cooked barley
- **Vegetables:** kale, lettuce, cauliflower, cucumber, broccoli, potatoes, wheat grass
- **Fruits:** ripe mangoes, pears, strawberries, watermelon

Neutral and balancing foods

These are the foods that are balancing to the body system at large. You can feed them with cooling foods or warming foods.

Specific neutral and balancing foods include:

bison	winter squash
cottage cheese	summer squash
cow's milk	zucchini
goat's milk	coconut
eggs (with yolk)	uncooked apples
flax	papayas
chia	blueberries
oats	camelina oil
carrots	almonds
pumpkin	sunflower seeds
sweet potatoes	

Feeding cooling, warming, and balancing foods

If it's summertime, and hot, and your dog has arthritis, you can add some cooling foods and neutral foods as part of a meal or as an entire meal. If your dog is less stiff in the summertime, stay with cooling and balancing foods. If your dog is stiff even in warm weather, blend warm and balancing foods for better circulation, as well as adding some cooling foods for reducing inflammation. You can make one meal cooling, and one meal warming. You can blend them. Your dog will tell you what foods works best for him/her.

In the case of GI tract inflammation like diarrhea, stay with cooling and balancing foods only. Likewise, if your dog gets cold easily, stay with warming foods.

Don't be afraid to combine neutral foods with cooling and warming foods. As you can see from the list, many wonderful foods for dogs are neutral and balancing!

Applying the principles of warming, cooling, and neutral foods can be tremendously beneficial if your dog has a health issue or is sensitive to seasonal temperatures. These principles are also helpful if your dog is active, and you need to cool the body system down after exertion.

As with all things food, listen to your intuition, don't be afraid of real food, and above all... listen to your dog.

Bovine Colostrum for Canines

Bovine colostrum is one of several superfoods for humans and canines. Its use goes back thousands of years to Ayurvedic medicine, although it came to be highlighted much more recently by members of the Australian swim team, who dominated the Olympic Games in 2000. Since then, athletes of various disciplines have used bovine colostrum to support healthy cellular replication and a robust immune system. But humans aren't the only ones who benefit from supplementing with this superfood. Bovine colostrum for dogs provides those signature benefits as well.

Growth Factors

Bovine colostrum contains over 70 different growth factors. These are responsible for supporting normal cellular repair and replication as well as DNA synthesis. The growth factors include:

- **Epidermal growth factor (EGF)**, which protects the skin, repairs cellular tissue
- **Insulin-like growth factors I & II**, which stimulate the repair and growth of DNA and RNA, and help to increase lean muscle mass
- **Transforming growth factors A & B**, which stimulate the proliferation of cells in connective

tissue and assist in the formation of bone and cartilage

Immune Factors

Bovine colostrum provides over 80 different immune factors including the **immunoglobulins**:

- **IgA**: one of the most prevalent antibodies produced by the immune system
- **IgG**: a specialized immune protein that responds to invasions of the lymphatic and circulatory system by bacteria, and viruses
- **IgM**: the first immunoglobulin produced when foreign substances like bacteria invade the body
- **IgE**: concentrated in the lungs, skin, and the cells of mucous membranes, providing the primary defense against environmental antigens

The immunoglobulins are the body's defense against invading pathogens.

Bovine colostrum also contains specific proline-rich polypeptides (PRPs) that regulate the thymus gland. PRPs can both stimulate a weakened immune system and balance an overactive immune system.

Cytokines: Interleukins, interferon, and lymphokines are components of bovine colostrum; these are chemicals that are involved in cell-to-cell communication and regulation of immune responses. Included among the many cytokines in bovine colostrum is *interleukin-10*, one of the most potent anti-inflammatory agents in the body.

Lactoferrin: A major component of bovine colostrum, this polyfunctional protein performs a vital function as part of the innate immune system, defending against pathogens including viruses. Lactoferrin also promotes the growth of the beneficial microorganism *Bifidobacteria*.

Transferrin: This is a mineral-binding carrier protein that can impede the growth of certain pathogenic bacteria, particularly in the gut.

Other nutritional elements

In addition to the components mentioned above, bovine colostrum includes probiotics, vitamins, minerals, glycoproteins, amino acids, and other nutritional factors. Colostrum also contains: the probiotic *Lactobacillus acidophilus*; macro- and micro-minerals including calcium, magnesium, phosphorus, potassium, sodium, copper, zinc, and selenium; specific amino acids L-taurine and L-carnitine; vitamins and antioxidants thiamine, riboflavin, vitamin E, vitamin A, and the antioxidant superoxide dismutase (SOD).

Benefits

- Dogs with allergies and other immune challenges benefit from the immunoglobulins, cytokines, and PRPs found in bovine colostrum.
- Dogs with gastrointestinal issues benefit from the growth factors in bovine colostrum, aiding mucosal repair.

- Senior dogs benefit both from the immune factors and growth factors in colostrum, supporting health and vitality.
- Performance dogs benefit from the immune support and the cellular repair activity, thus aiding in recovery.
- Dogs with connective tissue injuries benefit from the Transforming Growth Factors that stimulate cellular proliferation.

Bovine colostrum for dogs is not a panacea for all canine health issues. It is a whole food that complements the body's maintenance of homeostasis and wellness.

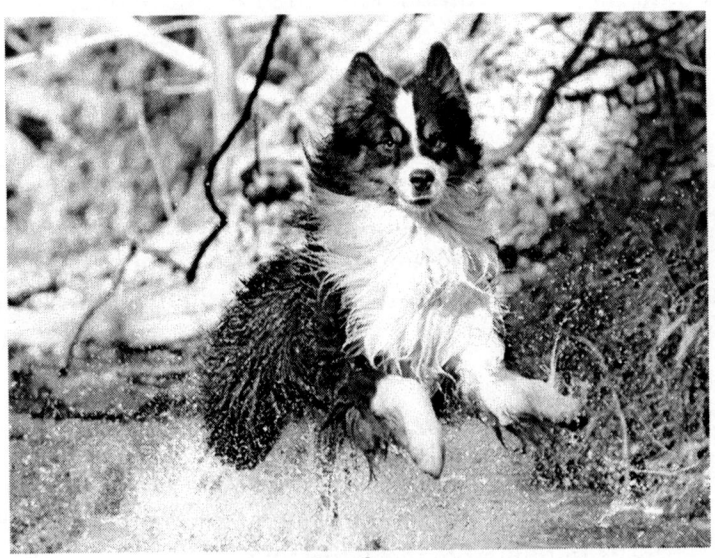

Crockett

Supplements

A healthy dog eating raw or home-cooked, or a combination that includes yogurt, lassi, or kefir should not need more supplementation than omega fatty acids and a whole-food multivitamin/mineral. Dogs that do not get live probiotics such as yogurt can benefit from supplemental live probiotic supplements.

Dogs that need to lose weight can benefit from supplementation with organic kelp, which helps speed up metabolism by supporting the thyroid.

Dogs with arthritis

Dogs with arthritis may benefit from glucosamine joint formulas. Personally, I've had zero success with a variety of canine joint supplement brands. I've had much better luck with bone broth and *Crominex 3+*. Found in BioStar's Juvenate K9 formula, Crominex 3+ is a patented blend of Indian gooseberry extract, shilajit, and chromium. This unique ingredient has been clinically studied to support healthy joints in dogs and supports healthy blood glucose levels and healthy endothelial function (Fleck et al., 2014).

I have found that results are not seen quickly with Crominex 3+ (it can take 60-90 days), but then the improvement in both soundness and pain is noticeable, and the longer the dog stays on it, the more significant the improvements.

Immune support

Dogs with immune issues including allergies do well with *bovine colostrum*. Dogs with connective tissue injuries also get important cellular support from the growth factors in colostrum. Certain mushrooms like *reishi* also provide immune support, as does coconut oil.

Turmeric and boswellia

Turmeric and boswellia provide antioxidant and anti-inflammatory actions in the body, particularly for muscle and joint strains. Turmeric offers powerful liver protection and helps to reduce toxins. There are dogs that won't eat turmeric or Boswellia sprinkled in their food. For these, try making "golden paste":

> ½ cup organic turmeric powder
> 1 to 1½ cups filtered water
> ½ teaspoon freshly ground black pepper
> ¼ cup organic coconut oil

> Mix turmeric with water in a pan (start with 1 cup of water and add more if needed). Stir on medium-low heat until a thick paste is formed (7-10 minutes). If your paste is watery, add more turmeric. Once you have paste, add the pepper and oil and stir well. Allow mixture to cool, then store in a glass jar with lid in the

refrigerator. Feed ¼ - ½ teaspoon several times per day. You can add the paste to your dog's food.

There is a powdered version of turmeric with ground black pepper and powdered coconut oil on the market called Turmericle from Stance Equine. It also includes the antioxidant *resveratrol*. If you don't want to make golden paste, this is an easy and very palatable alternative.

Calming supplements

There are many of these to choose from, and you might have to try several different kinds to see which one works best with your dog. With calming supplements in particular, one brand or formula does not work the same way on every dog.

My approach to calming is to deal with the stress that incites the anxiety, or over-reactiveness, or fear. I favor the herb *ashwaganda* because it regulates the stress hormone cortisol, and helps regulate the endocrine, circulatory, and glandular systems. *Holy basil* is another plant that regulates cortisol. Like ashwaganda, it helps to balance the body system. What I like about using these herbs is that they focus on the physiological aspects of stress by lowering cortisol production and bringing the body back to homeostasis.

Part III

Kemosabe's Point of View

Mealtime

One of the best times of the day is mealtime. It's the anticipation of delicious food, of course, but it's also our humans. They make mealtime fun.

Boss Lady says that preparing a meal is preparing medicine, and that the thoughts and feelings of the food preparer go into the food. A person who is angry or upset while preparing a meal will unknowingly be seasoning the food with those emotions. There is a rule at the farm that food for the animals is prepared with either a Zen calmness or happy, light-heartedness.

Peter likes to play the French Chef. He lets us into the kitchen speaking with a funny French accent and welcomes us to Chez Pierre's Bistro, "where Chef Pierre prepares for you a meal worthy of a star on the Champs-Élysées."

This gets the Aussie Tribe worked up. Crockett can barely stay in his skin. Peter describes each ingredient as he adds it to the bowls, increasing our excitement. Sometimes the Reverend Schmoo starts to salivate.

There are times when Peter likes to sing as he prepares our food. Boss Lady will join in, and then they are dancing around the kitchen, laughing, singing and we try to dance with them. Crockett, who has figured out how to howl, will join in vocally.

When Boss Lady does the meal preparation, she is either very quiet and calm and methodical, or she teases us saying, "This is the most incredible meal!" or "Oh my gosh, are you ready for this?" or "You are not going to *believe* how good this is!" Of course, we are beside ourselves. Not in a frantic way—in a tongue-hanging, tail-wagging (or in our case butt-wagging) way. You know...sort of like bursting with excitement but keeping it all inside.

Recently, Boss Lady has done most of the meal preparation because some of us got a little overweight on Chez Pierre's generous portions. He will walk into the kitchen while she's mixing up our food and say to the Reverend Mr. Schmoo, "I see Nurse Ratched has got you on a starvation diet," or "The Komandant has restricted your rations again." He will bend down and whisper, "You can always appeal to the Red Cross or the Geneva Convention."

This makes Boss Lady laugh, and in truth, we all do look less chunky on her regimen.

Personally, I think Peter is a bit of an Italian mother: hefty bowls of food signify love. The more food, the more love. The Reverend Mr. Schmoo and I, in particular, appreciate Peter's love food, but our long-term health is probably better served by Nurse Ratched's puritanical approach.

Mealtimes are generally between 6:00 and 6:30 a.m. and in the evening between 6:00 and 7:00. The evening meal is the most flexible, because Boss Lady can be working on something and then we have to remind her what time it is. Sometimes it's Thunderbear who lays his head on her lap while she's on the computer. Other times, I take the job of

Canine Mealtime Reminder and go sit beside her and give her my full-on grin.

"Okay, boys," she will say, "you'll just have to wait until I finish this."

That's when we send Crockett in for the kill. He woofs, he howls, he talks in a sing-song dog way, all the while standing next to Boss Lady's chair and staring at her. It never fails to work. "Oh, alright!" She gets up from her chair and we beat a path to the kitchen.

There are times when she has a meal plan all in her head, already worked out. There are other times she simply wanders around the kitchen murmuring utterances such as "Ummm" and "Hmmmm." Then she will perk up and start arranging foods on the counter: "...and maybe some of this, and I think you guys would love to have a little of this..."

The Reverend whispers, "I'll take anything that is edible."

The nice thing about mealtime is that we don't have to go out and hunt and kill for a meal. Besides, this have-the-human-provide-all-vittles arrangement is immensely practical because we canines are all paws in the kitchen.

Bison for Breakfast

As a canine living with a whole food nutritionist, I am fortunate to get a variety of foods to eat: raw, cooked, and sometimes a mixture of both with assorted vegetables and fruits. Luckily, none of us in the Aussie Tribe are food sensitive or have particularly delicate GI tracts. My favorite meat of all is raw bison. That is the most delicious food on the planet and, according to my human, one of the best foods for dogs.

Bison are always free-ranged because they don't fit in most barns, and they get grumpy and aggressive if humans try to make them behave like cows. Bison eat a wider range of grasses than cattle.

At 2.42 grams of fat per 100 grams, bison meat is much lower in fat than beef (9.28 g), pork (9.21 g), or chicken (7.41 g). This is important for dogs who have spreading waistlines and those of us who want to maintain a healthy weight but still want to eat great food.

Ground bison provides 22 grams of protein per 3 ounces. This is four times what an egg provides and one gram more than the same-sized serving of ground beef. Bison also provides as many omega-3s per serving as salmon, and 3-6 times the amount of omega-3s as grain-fed animals. Bison meat is one of the richest sources of CoQ10, which is required by cells to produce energy and help protect the body from free-radical damage.

Bison are not injected with growth hormones, antibiotics or other drugs and chemicals. For one thing, bison are cranky and don't like to be messed with. Secondly, the National Bison Association passed a resolution opposing the use of these substances in the production of bison for meat.

Ground bison can be found at Whole Foods and other health food grocery stores. You can cook it like hamburger, or feed it raw. I like raw best because it is a lot like eating live prey— similar to squirrels I've caught, which I don't often get to chew on because the humans take them away.

My human says that raw ground bison provides improved nutrient assimilation because the food enzymes are still alive, and haven't been cooked out. Because our bodies can utilize raw meat so well, there is less poop for our human to pick up. But I like bison because it tastes great. Maybe it connects me back to my ancestors, the wolves, who hunted and dined on bison. Maybe it connects me to food that has a bit of the wild in it, and that speaks to the wild in all canines.

Lassi (not Lassie)

Okay, so I know that Lassie is some famous collie dog that the humans get all soft and mushy about as soon as they hear the name. Well I can tell you that we Aussies get pretty soft-eyed and wiggly when we hear the same magic word: *lassi*. Well, it sounds the same. And it's almost as delicious as a dehydrated liver treat.

Lassi is a traditional fermented drink of the Punjab region of India, made from yogurt and water, sometimes with salt or spices added. It dates back thousands of years, and is a well-known Ayurvedic beverage for GI tract health, which makes it an excellent probiotic treat for us canines.

The brand of lassi that we get has not been homogenized. This is important because the purpose of homogenization is to break down fat molecules in milk so they resist separation—no cream rising to the top, so to speak. Because it is not homogenized, my human has to shake the bottle really well. Sometimes she does this while singing: "Shake, Shake, Shake, Shake Your Booty." It's kind of fun to watch your human gyrating at the sink, singing a silly song. Of course, what we Aussies want to know is, what's a booty?

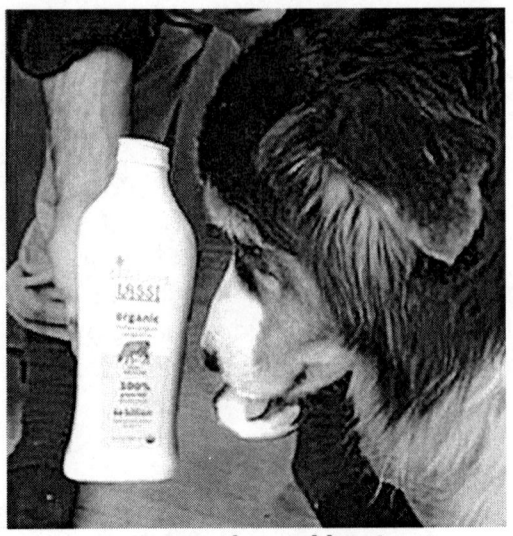

Kemosabe and lassi

According to our human, lassi is a balancing probiotic for all three of Ayurvedic medicine's body types: **vata** (air), **pitta** (fire), and **kapha** (water and earth). Due to its heavy nature, it pacifies the air of *vata*; because of its cooling properties, it balances the fire of *pitta*; and, because no sugar is added, it is balancing to the water and earth of *kapha*.

Lassi can be mixed into a meal, but we love it so much that we're always happy to just lick from a big spoon! Whatever drops on the floor, Crockett vacuums up. He is pretty convenient to have around for floor cleaning.

The difference between kefir and lassi

We also get *kefir* as an alternative probiotic. Lassi contains several strains of bacteria, while kefir contains more—up to 36 different microorganisms. Also, the fermentation process differs between these two probiotics. Lassi is fermented with bacteria only, while kefir is fermented with bacteria and yeast.

Because kefir contains yeast cultures, it can be heating to the GI tract. If one of us has diarrhea, we won't get kefir, we will get lassi. Sometimes our human mixes lassi with organic pumpkin meal if our stools are too loose. The pumpkin gives us more fiber, and the lassi is cooling to the GI tract. Likewise, when Buckaroo's GI tract slows down and his stool is a little hard, he gets kefir to add more heat to the digestive system.

Our human believes in rotating probiotics; some days it's good to get kefir, some days it's good to get lassi. We also get a premium probiotic supplement once or twice a week that contains microorganisms specific to the canine GI tract. She just sprinkles it in our food, and those microorganisms go straight to where they're needed most.

Aliens Among Us

Forget the old sci-fi flicks about aliens in flying saucers. Forget E.T. and Area 51. Aliens are here now, and they have been on this planet for a very long time. They are called cats. And frankly, I wish they would phone home or get beamed up and leave Earth to the canines.

First of all, they are sneaky. Not in a clever, smart-dog way, but in a conniving, not-to-be-trusted alien way. They are stealth creatures with hidden knives in their paws. I think when they first landed on Earth thousands of years ago, they must have landed in the Far East, because they have become ninjas and *kung-fu* masters.

Their alien nature makes them spit, hiss, and cough up hairballs, which is really disgusting. And no wonder they cover up their poo...that's an alien stench if I ever smelled one.

There are two aliens in the house: Sumo, the cat the size of a small country at 24 pounds, and the long-haired black cat Sooty, aka The Bowling Ball—so named because when I was a puppy, I sort of skidded into him while he was napping on the floor and we both slid for a few feet and he ended up slammed into the coffee table, causing a tower of magazines to fall. Strike!

The mission of the aliens is to control their living space and surrounding environs as well as the other creatures in it: bugs, birds, rodents, squirrels, dogs, horses, and humans. One of the horses tried to nuzzle the Bowling Ball off of the paddock fence and was immediately met by Bruce Lee armed with daggers. Boy, was that horse surprised.

Humans, being human, are the most easily manipulated; a meow or a trill and the human is emotional toast. Or the alien turns on The Purr. You see The Purr is a very unique alien feature that exploits humans. The science of The Purr is that it has a peak 220-520-hertz frequency range, and human baby cries are in a similar range: 330-600 hertz. The Purr also has lower frequencies of 14-140 vibrations per second that are therapeutic for pain relief, bone growth, and healing...for the cat. This of course totally explains the "nine lives" phenomenon; the aliens have an advanced way of self-healing.

A good example of cat manipulation of humans is food. When Sumo or Sooty are hungry, they meow, sometimes combined with a purr for extra exploitation, coupled with a feline body- wrap around the human's legs. Suddenly the human is all, "Oh, are you hungry? Let me get you some food."

Now, if we canines bark, or get excited over the prospect of food, or if I walk over and smile at my human with the old "I'm hungry" look, the response I get is, "It's not dinner time yet, go lie down."

Dogs are on a schedule. Cats do as they please.

And I would like to know why aliens like boxes and paper bags. You'd think because they are aliens they come from a more advanced society, but the evidence is clear: amusing oneself by crawling into a box or a Whole Foods paper sack isn't enlightened...it's deranged.

Chasing cats is strictly *verboten* at our house. Chasing a cat can land a dog behind bars: the ever-unpopular dog gates that restrict us to one room in the house. And while the cats lounge on the couch in the living room, I sit behind wooden bars watching the aliens monopolize the humans. Just call me the Prisoner of Zenda.

I used to wonder what my human sees in cats, why she shares our space with them. Then I realized that my human is a victim of a cunning alien race that has enslaved humanity. Thank goodness we canines are here to offset this feline manipulation, to stand against the possibility of cat domination, to keep the songbirds safe and do what the aliens cannot do: protect, serve, and bark.

Living with Cats

There are basically four kinds of humans in the world: those living with dogs, those living with cats, those living with dogs and cats, and those living without dogs or cats. This advice is for the dogs living with humans who also live with cats.

First of all, humans think that when cats meow, it is a way of saying *"I love you."* That couldn't be further from the truth. When a cat meows, it means one of three things: *I'm hungry, clean the litter box,* or *put the dog outside for my comfort and convenience.* When a cat meows to a dog, the message is: *I am only being nice to you because the human is watching.*

Among all the insults experienced when you're living with cats, there is nothing more humiliating than having the resident cat rub up against you, marking his "territory". Humans think this is *so cute*, and that somehow the cat really loves the dog. HA. As soon as the human is out of earshot, the cat gives the dog a good swipe across the nose, or maybe even the most disgusting gesture of all: running its tail under the dog's chin or chest. ICK. Time to head for a horse water trough, or have a good roll in the dirt.

Some of the most fun that dogs can have living with felines is by playing a game called "Chase the Cat." Very invigorating. Unfortunately, in our house where the cats are the size of small countries, they don't run very fast. When I am at a barn, and I see a barn cat, I just want to run as fast as I can and chase that cat into a tree. I don't want to hurt the cat, or eat the cat (yuck). It's simply a demonstration of the superior power of canines. Of course there are the very smart cats, who, upon seeing a dog, just lie down and flick their tails in anticipation of the cat-paw-knife-strike on the nose. Take it from me, those can really hurt.

At our house we also like to play "Blame the Cat." This can only happen when the human is outside or away from the home. Whenever Thunderbear pulls food off the kitchen counter, or I mistakenly drop one of my human's shoes in the dog water bowl, or Buckaroo climbs into the *forbidden chair*, or Crockett unrolls the toilet paper roll and runs through the house flinging bits of toilet paper everywhere.... that's the time to play this game. When the human walks in, we sit innocently in front of her and let her know it wasn't us. It was the *cat*.

I find one of the most annoying things about living with cats is that they are bed hogs. If one or both cats are in the human's bed before we get there, trying to dislodge them is like trying to dislodge a log with claws. These cats don't move. And they get very bent out of shape when Buckaroo tries to encourage their departure from *our bed* by jumping as close to them as possible without landing on them. They scratch us, they claw us, they hiss at us, they make ugly throat noises. We have found that if all four of us jump on the bed at the same time, the cats will eventually depart in a sulky way.

Of course, it is not just the human's bed either. One bowling ball of a cat likes to sleep on our deluxe West Paw dog beds, and knead the lovely soft cover with his needle claws because he's too lazy to go outside and scratch a fence post. We try to get him to move by barking as loudly as we can into his ears. Then, of course, the human comes and rescues him. And as she picks him up, he gives us that look: *neener neener neener.*

Living with cats. It's a weird kind of canine karma, I think.

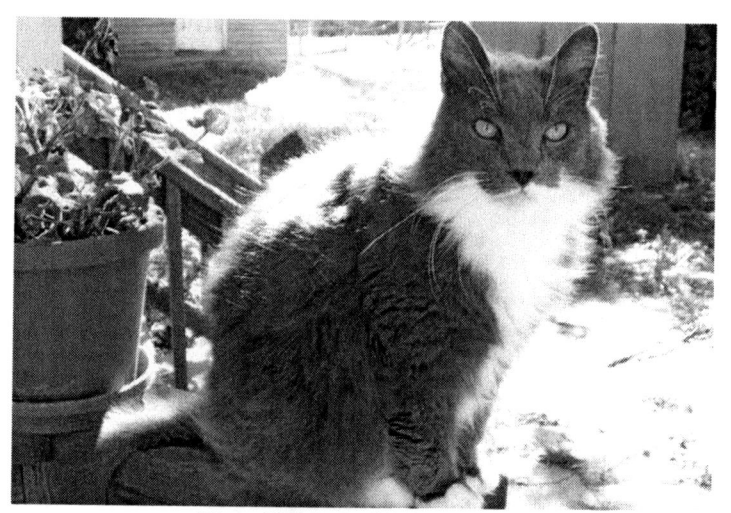

King Henry of Springdale

On the Road Again

Every January, we pack up and head to the Winter Equestrian Festival in Wellington, Florida. I, of course, must travel with Boss Lady as her protector, companion, and anxiety-reducer. It's not easy.

This year Crockett is coming too. He is annoying in a youngest-dog-of-the-pack way, but I've taught him how to be a good traveler: no puking, or whining, or hogging the back seat. Bark only if Boss Lady is attacked or threatened. Barking at semi trucks is fruitless and will make a dog hoarse.

Our human always has reams of lists full of reminders of what to pack. Problem is, she will get up in the middle of the night to write something down that she doesn't want to forget, and leave it in a place like on the back of the toilet, or under a book, and then later dash madly about trying to find that scrap of paper. It really is quite amusing, especially this year, when that piece of paper was found on her bed, under a cat.

The first day of the two-day drive to Florida is the longest. We are subjected to various rock CDs, satellite radio pop stations, and ultimately a book on tape. Boss Lady likes biographies, and I have learned a lot over the years about Ted Kennedy, Billy Crystal, Johnny Carson, Steve Jobs, and two dudes called Lewis and Clark who went on a big walkabout, starving, having to carry their canoes, and ended up discovering America.

Boss Lady has never met a speed limit sign she agrees with, so from our place in the back seat it feels a lot like we are traveling at warp speed. She also likes the left lane. Spirit Dog told me once that the left lane is for burning gasoline as quickly as possible so that the human can get to a rest stop or gas station quickly. I do wonder—if Boss Lady's bladder was larger, would we drive in the right lane and stop less often?

Gas stations are strange places. They have interesting food smells mingling with the toxic fumes of petroleum. Boss Lady is quick to point out that the greasy, fat dripping scents are not *edible* food smells, which translates into: we aren't getting any of that food. Out come the leashes and we are expected to get our business done in nanoseconds. I have long resisted this notion, preferring to sniff as many bushes, blades of grass, and previous canine calling cards as possible. Crockett, however, is weak. Show him a patch of grass and he lifts his leg instantly.

The most fun thing about driving to Wellington is the motel. We generally spend the first night around Savannah, in some cheap hotel off I-95. I generally can scare the bejesus out of the construction workers and send a few kids screaming with my seriously deep bark. Of course there are those motel guests who see me and say, "Oh what a beautiful dog," so I turn on my trademark Aussie charm, complete with smile.

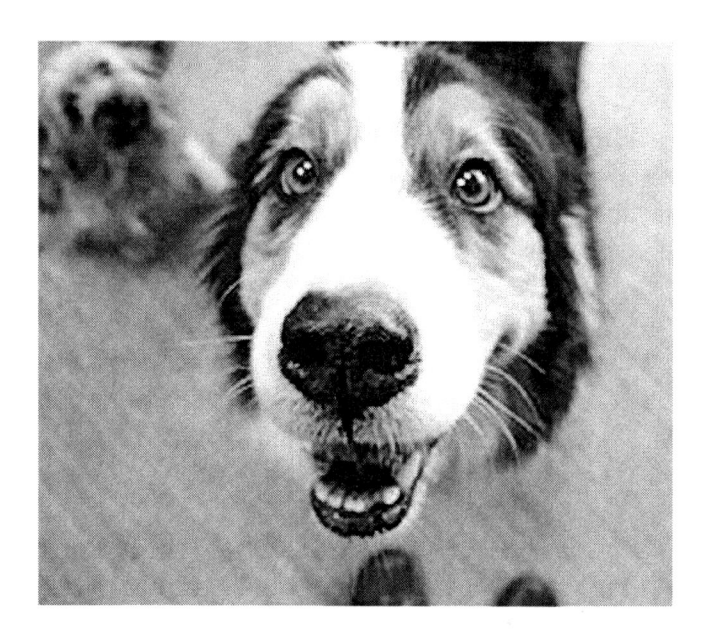

In the motel room, I lie up against the outside door to make sure no one comes in. I have learned not to growl at the sound of footsteps on the pavement outside, or at the sound of a diesel starting up at 4 a.m. Boss Lady can get cranky.

One time I was traveling with Thunderbear and Buckaroo, who was only four months old at the time. We were coming back up from Florida, and stopped at a motel for the night. Boss Lady went out to get some dinner. We got bored. Thunderbear thought it would be fun to jump from bed to bed, and then grabbed a pillow and we had a pillow fight. Buckaroo grabbed the bed spread and pulled it off with my help. Boss Lady walked into the room and nearly had a massive heart attack. She later described the incident like this: "Imagine a slumber party of adolescent boys in your motel room…"

Since we are fed predominantly raw food, a cooler travels with us that plugs into an outlet in the Subaru and in the motel room to keep things cool. We always get a raw marrow- bone to eat after we have finished our regular raw food patties. This keeps us occupied and amused while our human lies comatose on the bed.

When we get to Wellington, before even going to the rental house, we stop at the dog park so that we can blow off some steam after being cooped up in the car and walked on leashes. Ah, the freedom to sniff, and roll, and run. It's not home, but it will do.

When we get to the rental house, I have to check things out, sniff out any possible varmints in the fenced yard, observe Boss Lady lugging in all the suitcases, computer, and paraphernalia she must have, and then I make sure she grabbed The Dog Bag and the portable cooler. After this kind of trip, we need food, a little time in the backyard, and a long peaceful sleep on a carpet that doesn't move at 80 miles an hour.

Tips for humans on driving long distances with canines:

- Don't forget the food.
- Pack paper towels…just in case.
- Tell us how wonderful we are throughout the trip, not just when you have successfully avoided a collision with a tractor-trailer.
- Maintain your sense of humor. If you don't have one, order one from Amazon before you leave on your trip.

- Don't curse when you miss an exit or turn the wrong way. Our mothers taught us not to say bad things, and we are embarrassed when you do.

Rescue Me

It has finally happened: I am in Dog Hell.

The humans rescued a little terrier mix that was running down the middle of the road. At first I thought, well, how nice and compassionate my humans are. After the little tyke is fed and taken care of, she can go live somewhere else.

But she's still here. She is bossy, dictatorial, and possessive. She thinks she owns the couch. So far she has bitten Crockett on the foot: boy was he surprised, chased Thunderbear out of the room, sent Buckaroo into "time out", and actually challenged me for the premier back-seat car space.

She *was* going to go live with Boss Lady's mother in Arizona...but she has all these canine health problems that make her unsuitable. I can tell you it's not just her immune system problems, or her stinky skin, or all the medicines and treatments and special foods that make her unsuitable. It's her dominating personality and rule-the-roost attitude. Where does a dog weighing a mere 13 pounds get off telling me what to do?

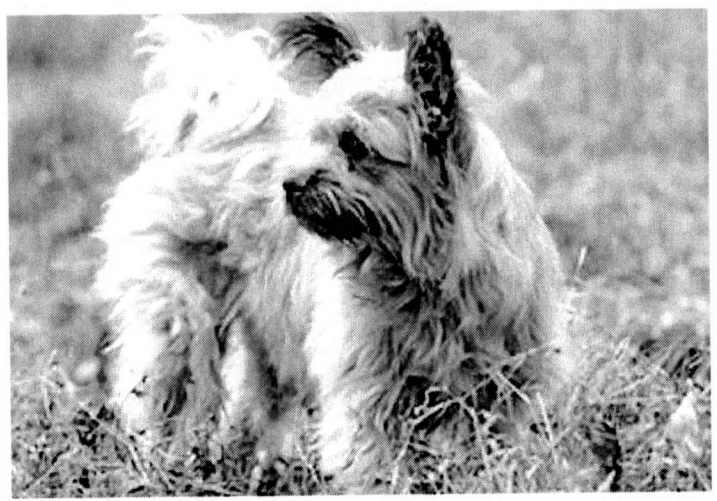

Yoda, the terrible terrier

Normally small dogs bow down to me (with the exception of Pomeranians who just pretend I'm invisible). Small dogs accept my authority and my size; after all, I can body slam as well as Hulk Hogan. Small dogs can be fun to play with, especially if they run fast so I can chase them like squirrels. This small dog, however, is some kind of a terrorist clearly sent here to disrupt my kingdom and usurp my throne. On top of that, she has attached herself to Boss Lady like a fuzzy brown tick. Not only is she needy, she is high maintenance.

To make matters worse, the humans have given her a *name*, and a collar, which in the dog world means: she isn't leaving. Boss Lady calls her *Yoda*, which is odd, because I've sat beside Boss Lady and watched and re-watched those Star Wars movies more times than I've caught squirrels, and I can tell you that this terrier is nothing like Jedi Master Yoda.

First of all she can't levitate, or take her paw and raise an X-wing starfighter out of a swamp, let alone our pond. She wouldn't know a lightsaber from a flashlight or a Wookie from a Newfie.

As you might imagine, we Aussies have been a bit stressed over this overbearing, thinks-she's-our-empress dog in our midst. Luckily, our human has been working on a canine stress formula and we have been among the test dogs used for the various batches. Let me tell you...those little tasty treats are like *magic*. At a higher dose, it's like having the best nap ever in the world. Even at a low dose, the terrier interloper doesn't annoy me. No matter how hard she barks or how imperious she gets, I couldn't care less. Here's what's even better: when the terrier is given one of the stress treats, there is peace in the kingdom for many hours.

Of course, the stress treats don't solve all of our problems...like finally getting the bossy little terrier to head on down the road. Can't we just trade her for another Australian shepherd, or a couple of packages of marrow bones?

Yoda has lived with us for a year now, and yesterday she left with her new humans: a mother and daughter who live in another state. She is going to be an ONLY dog, which suits her royal highness, and her new humans have already picked out clothes for her; would love to know if she gets a tiara.

Peace has descended once again. Thunderbear and Crockett are back sharing the couch, I don't have to take a wide berth around the coffee table, and the Reverend Mr. Schmoo has returned to his place on the floor next to the couch. I think the cats miss Yoda, though. They liked to take swipes at her fanny and steal food out of her food bowl. Yes, the cats will miss her. Me, and the tribe...not so much.

Skunked

My human says it's some kind of miracle: I have gone a whole year without getting skunked by a skunk. I do have the honorable distinction of being the only member of the Aussie tribe to be skunked. It is another reason I am special. However, there was one dog who lived at the farm during Spirit and Rocky Raccoon's time, named Rutrow, who got skunked several times each summer.

Rutrow was another one of Boss Lady's rescues, and looked like a large version of a Walt Disney Dog. Honestly, he looked like an 80-pound overgrown mop. And he loved cats. He let them sleep with him, curl up under his chin and cozy up to him on cold winter nights. Personally, I think he must have been some kind of weirdo.

Rutrow thought that skunks were kitties, so he got skunked at least two or three times per year—right in the face of course, and in all that hair, which resulted in gagging reflexes from the human, Rutrow's banishment from the house, and the subsequent tomato juice bath procedure. The tomato juice on a cream-colored hairy mop dog made him look like a character from a slasher film: *Rutrow on Elm Street*. He generally needed two tomato juice applications several hours apart to begin to reduce the skunk's odiferous odor. And even despite two applications, the lingering undertones of skunk remained for weeks, as did a lightly pink tinge to his facial hair.

When I first got skunked, it was on my chest of thick, white double-coated hair. Boss Lady decided on apple cider vinegar diluted with two parts water. I was glad to be spared the tomato juice routine, but the vinegar didn't quite get all the skunk smell out. In fact, when I went swimming in the pond several days later, the skunk odor once again wafted from my chest, prompting my human to scoop up handfuls of mud-clay from the bank of the creek, and slather my chest with the dark ooze. Her theory was that the clay-mud would bind to what she referred to as "toxic odors". She let the clay-mud dry, kept me out of the house for a few hours, and then washed me. This technique was moderately successful, but as she leaned down and smelled my chest, her nose detected a lingering odor.

So she did what any woman with a war chest of essential oils and potions does: she rubbed essential oil of frankincense and myrrh into my coat. I smelled like a Gift of the Magi for quite a while.

The following spring I got skunked again, this time on my nose and forehead. My human started her requisite gagging, ushering me back out the door I had just come in from. Her remedy this time was something she found with Google: 1 quart hydrogen peroxide, ¼ cup baking soda, and 1 teaspoon dishwashing liquid. Of course this was more than she needed to do just my face, but in her waste-not-want-not philosophy, she decided to apply it to my legs, chest, and back as well.

She rubbed the mixture in while I stood stoically and Spirit lay on his back laughing. She didn't have rubber gloves, which the recipe called for, so she went to the barn and got a pair of equine disposable fecal exam gloves, which quite honestly looked like they belonged to Paul Bunyan. She rinsed me thoroughly, washed me in one of her herbal shampoos, rinsed me again, and then toweled me off.

I had had quite enough of this, despite my immense patience and the fact that now I smelled a bit like a department store's fragrance counter. As soon she unsnapped my leash, I was off, thinking about a nice equine manure pile to roll in but stopping instead at the grass-less area beneath the old walnut tree, for a good body-to-earth gyration in the dirt.

You might be wondering, why is it that I repeatedly get skunked year after year? Look, I am a herding dog. Anything that moves that isn't human is within my natural instincts to *drive, move along, put the pedal to the metal, you're outta here.* I don't have anything personally against skunks or squirrels or foxes or raccoons or possums or deer. I just need to send them on their way, make them acquiesce to my will, make them scamper away in fear of my Awesome Aussie-ness.

Let me just say that skunks don't like to be herded, especially not the little ones, the kits, who don't control their spray as well as an adult skunk does. These little critters are easily startled, so they tend to let loose their chemical smelliness often.

Adult skunks can spray over a distance of ten feet. How do I know this? I was a good ten feet away the fourth time I got nailed by a skunk. I thought I was safe and I barked at her to get out of Dodge, and she turned around and sprayed me, which is the skunk equivalent of *Hey, you, get off of my cloud.*

Now that I've gone a year being skunk-free—while getting *no* extra treats for this accomplishment I might add—I will let you in on a secret: the reason I haven't been skunked is that they all moved to a neighbor's shed down the road.

The Puppy Cometh

Well, my human did it again and brought another puppy into the pack. I have endured three puppies already: Thunderbear, Buckaroo, and Crockett. Now there's a new one: Wookie. And to top it off, she's a girl.

Here's the thing about puppies: they aren't really dogs yet. They're more like live squeaky toys who can't control their bladders. The good thing about puppies is that their attention span is about the same as a gnat's, which makes stealing their toys infinitely easy. They also sleep a lot, which the human appreciates.

My fellow pack members' initial reactions to Wookie ranged from long-suffering (Thunderbear), to "she doesn't exist in my Universe" (Buckaroo), to Crockett's "I'm not touching it, it might have cooties." This is fairly amusing to the human, because Crockett is an intact male and he will probably sing a different song when Wookie goes into season. Since I essentially raised my younger pack members, I've again taken on my usual role as Nanny Dog and Hall Monitor to Wookie, teaching her the rules of pack life and the hierarchy.

Wookie came from the same breeder as the rest of the pack, so she had been on a free-feed kibble program. Free-feed means that the kibble is available to the puppy all the time. The first thing the human did was start a feeding schedule:

small meals four times per day. Wookie gets the kibble she was weaned on, plus a little raw food mixed in. Eventually she will transition to all raw, and twice-a-day meals. But right now, at 10 weeks of age, the human thinks small meals more often are better for her GI tract, and more of what she is used to having since she was raised on free-feed.

Wookie will start on a whole-food multivitamin supplement powder to cover all the vitamin and mineral requirements of a growing puppy. As far as treats, she has been introduced to whole-food liver treats (broken into little pieces) along with small bits of dehydrated liver. So far she's a lot like Buckaroo: she hasn't met a food she hasn't liked. Of course, the human is keeping her away from things like fresh horse manure (one of the pack's favorites), and she's not big enough to reach the cat food bowls on the table, which are one of my favorite illicit snacks. Nor has she been introduced to Thunderbear's egg-stealing missions but that will certainly come in time.

This puppy qualifies as a piranha, but at this age she needs stuff to chew on that doesn't include the human's slippers, electrical cords, the leather couch, a cell phone, or my fur. Our human goes to a specialty dog store and gets these bully stick rings that are easy for the puppy to hold in her paws and gnaw on. Our human also buys dehydrated chicken feet for the puppy to chew. Often the puppy will fall asleep after she has had a time of vigorous chewing, and then I slip in, quiet as a mouse, and steal the chew. It is one of the perks of being the Hall Monitor.

Our human has already begun clicker training, which she did with all of us when we were pups. Next month, Wookie will go to puppy class like we did. Puppy class is a good way for Wookie to meet other puppies and socialize in a safe setting. It also helps our human to remember training tips she has forgotten due to her advanced age and all, but don't tell her I said that.

Friends of our human ask, how is it that the pack gets along with a new puppy. My response: it's all about how the human approaches it. Our human didn't stress about introducing Wookie to the pack, didn't come up with fear scenarios in her head, or expect discord within the pack. She introduced us one at a time to Wookie and then we all got treats. She makes sure every day that each member of the pack gets plenty of attention and that our routine stays the same, despite Wookie's presence.

The benefits of a new puppy in the house are the toys. All these new toys show up, which is great for me, because I like to steal them from under Wookie's nose. Maybe it's not as James Bond-ian as Thunderbear's egg-stealing escapades, but for an older dog such as myself...it's the little things.

Tigger Montague

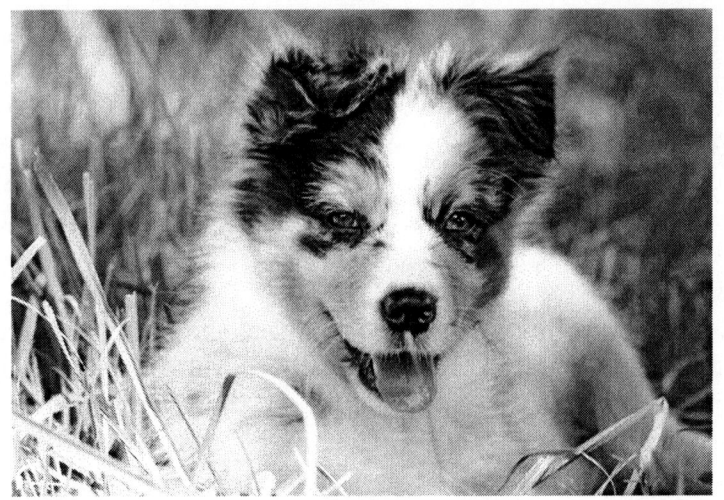

Wookie

When Bad Stress Happens to Good Dogs

The benefits we canines have of sharing our lives with humans include love and companionship and good food. Since I was a puppy, I have always appreciated that my human is my own personal concierge. But one of the challenges we canines face when we share our lives with humans is dealing with human stress. We feel it; not just in our bodies and our minds, but in our hearts. It hurts us to see our humans in distress.

There have only been a very few times that I have seen Boss Lady just fall apart from stress—what we dogs call *Human Extreme Meltdown*. This is quite a bit different from regular human meltdown, expressed as frustration, anger, weeping, and hurtling curse words at supersonic speed. Human Extreme Meltdown is expressed as crawling under the covers in a fetal position, immediately followed by hyperactivity, insomnia, frantic cleaning while chanting swear words in unique and original combinations, and spontaneously bursting into tears while crawling back into fetal position under a blanket. All I can do when Boss Lady gets like this is stay right beside her, telling her *"It's going to be okay."*

During one particularly stressful event, her anguish was so intense that she sounded like a wounded animal with its leg caught in a trap. I was very worried, and my stomach got upset, and I couldn't figure out what to do. I tried bringing her my favorite toys so that she might want to carry one around in her mouth like I do. I brought her my Frisbee so that she would have something fun to play with. I licked her face and her hands, like my dog friends do for me. But nothing seemed to work. Her stress was from betrayal. We canines don't experience betrayal among our own kind; betrayal is a distinctly human affliction that we don't really understand.

We all tried our best to help our human. Thunderbear kept dropping twigs and sticks in Boss Lady's lap, telling her it was a great chill pill. "Just gnaw on this and you'll feel lots better," he told her.

Spirit Dog attempted many times to coax her into meditation, by lying on his back with all four feet in the air, his eyes closed in bliss, in his classic Australian shepherd Zen mode.

Nothing worked. Her stress encompassed me like an extra fur coat. I didn't know how to get rid of it until, finally, my GI tract did it for me.

There is something about raging diarrhea in a dog that can motivate a human into action. Boss Lady began to compile her concoction:

- **holy basil**, an herb that helps reduce cortisol elevated by stress
- **fermented lassi**, a cooling live probiotic
- **kaolin clay**, which helps bind toxins
- **organic pumpkin meal**, a good source of fiber.

She mixed it all together and added it to my food. By the following day, my GI tract was headed back towards normal.

While I express chronic stress through my GI tract, other dogs experience stress in different ways. Thunderbear goes anorexic, losing all appetite except for treats. Spirit Dog always went in the opposite direction; he ate anything and everything in his path including, but not limited to, cat poop, freshly-caught moles, a stick of butter left on the counter, or anything he could con Peter into sharing, such as peanut-butter-and-banana sandwiches, veggie burgers, or vanilla ice cream.

It appears that when some humans are in stress meltdown, they miss the signs of stress in their dogs until one of us exhibits stress in a smelly way that's not to be missed. Then there are humans in stress meltdown who become even more hyper-vigilant, as if everything happening is a disaster. Neither one of these scenarios is optimal for the canines. It would help us a lot if you could go take a walk with us in the forest, or play catch, or take us for a ride in the car, or just let go and let us be beside you, helping you heal.

Tigger Montague

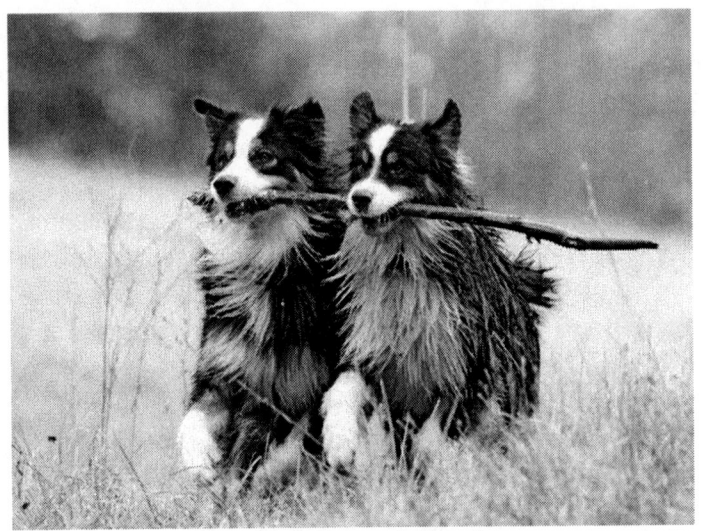

Thunderbear and Crockett

Canine Tips for Happy Holidays

We dogs know that after the Day of the Turkey, things can get a little crazy in the human world until the day of the new year when normalcy begins to return. Humans can get a little uptight, stressed, frantic or depressed during the holidays, so it is up to us to help them out. A few things to remember during this time of year:

The Christmas tree

It is so thoughtful of humans to put a tree in the house and decorate it for the cats. I don't know why it's not called a Catmas tree. Last year Buckaroo tried herding the cats around the tree, causing one cat to climb it, which sent these little glass orbs crashing to the floor. Need I say the human was not pleased? Also, the tree is not for emergency urination or for leaving a message to another dog in the household.

The wrapping paper

Those long rolls of brightly colored paper are not for playing tug of war, or bashing another dog in the head. Humans use this to cover the surprises in the boxes that they shriek over. Little children are especially good at shrieking when they rip open a wrapped gift. *Do not panic;*

the child is not in danger. Most importantly, do not grab the toy that was in the box and run off with it, thinking you are saving the child. This causes wailing from the child at the decibel level of a siren, and the adults will launch themselves like missiles off the couch to get the toy away from you.

The Food

There are lots of tasty, yummy things around during the holidays. I particularly like the little gobs of almond cookie batter that occasionally hit the floor, and the crumbs that fall from the human eating a gingerbread bar. Do not eat the dark cookies or the cookies with dark little chips in them; that is called *shocklate* and the humans call it that because, if we dogs eat it, we will go into shock and it may be too late. I have heard tell of a black lab who ate a box of *shocklate*-covered cherries and then proceeded to have raging diarrhea all over the house. Humans really don't like cleaning up diarrhea, particularly from their favorite carpets. It is a testament to that Labrador's sturdy GI tract that she was no worse for wear.

The eggnog

Thunderbear discovered eggnog due to his incredible balance, standing on his hind legs with his front paws on the counter. He managed to knock over a carton of it, which spilled to the floor, and which we all happily lapped up until the human walked in. It is best to avoid consuming eggnog, as most humans add rum and cognac to it. This makes the humans very happy, but we canines don't hold our liquor well.

The plants

Don't eat poinsettias, mistletoe, or holly no matter how hungry you are, or what the cats say. You *can*, of course, rip a few leaves off the poinsettias and just leave them on the floor and blame it on the cats.

Santa Paws

This is the Big Dog that brings dog toys and puts them under the tree, or in a stocking that hangs from the fireplace mantle. The humans say Santa Paws gets driven around town by reindeer and he gets very hungry, so they leave a plate of cookies for him. **Do not eat the cookies**, or Santa Paws will leave medicine in your stocking instead of a marrow bone.

Food for the Holidays

It's that time of year when we canines start smelling all the yummy aromas coming out of the kitchen. You know...the cookies, breads, pies, and the crumbs that fall on the floor and must be immediately cleaned up by the Aussie Tribe. We call it floor polishing.

It's easy for humans to fall prey to our pleading eyes and soulful expressions in the kitchen. They'll sneak us food under the dinner table or share a snack with us, or even leave some delicious cheese out on the counter. But a lot of what humans eat is not good for us, no matter how adept we are at begging.

So, every year we get a special Christmas breakfast stew that is nourishing, delicious, and good for us. Buckaroo may say that he'd prefer a couple of gingerbread cookies, but when the crockpot lid is opened on Christmas morning, we are all drooling for our special meal. Now, without further ado:

Kemosabe's Christmas Stew

1. Line bottom of crockpot with marrow bones and chicken wings. Add roast or a steak or venison. Add water almost up to the top.
2. Add 4 tablespoons organic apple cider vinegar (to help draw out the minerals from the marrow bones.)

3. Add 1/3 cup split peas and 1-2 sweet potatoes, sliced or quartered. You can also add sliced carrots and celery.
4. Cook on low for 10-12 hours. Our human does this at night, so by morning we have stew.
5. Remove and discard the marrow bones after cooking. Debone the chicken wings and discard. Never feed cooked bones to dogs!
6. Add about ¼ cup chopped kale to the crockpot and stir. Allow stew to cool for at least a half hour.
7. Cut the meat and divide it among the dog bowls. Pour the vegetables/potatoes and broth over the meat. Our human adds a tablespoon or two of *lassi* or *kefir* to each bowl to make it creamier and to provide some good probiotics.
8. Add 1-2 tablespoons of organic pumpkin meal for added fiber. Mix well.

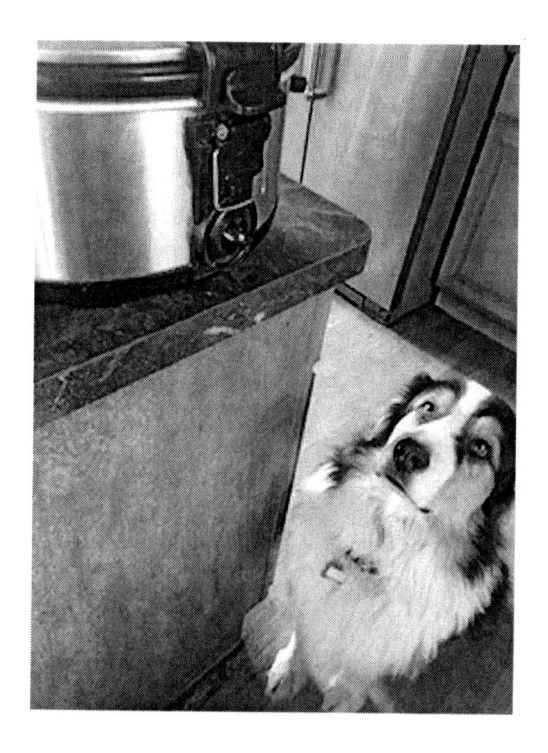

Voila!—a healthy, nutrient-dense meal that you can't get out of a bag or a can...or from a human's Christmas cookie.

A few more things to consider:

- If you currently feed raw, just make the broth with the vegetables and sweet potatoes and pour over the raw food.
- Or make bone broth.
- You can also substitute the marrow -bones with chicken necks, and put chicken breasts or thighs or a combination on top.

- When the stew is done, make sure to discard the bones in a place where we canines can't find them or dig them out.
- Lastly, set your watch, because your dog will consume this delicious Christmas Stew in nanoseconds. Thankfully, there will be no leftovers for the cats.

Appendix A: Home-Cooked Recipes

I like to cook meals in a crockpot on the low setting, either overnight or all day long if I'm at work. With the following recipes, make sure to add plenty of water—enough to cover the ingredients by one or two inches. If you're like me and sometimes forget to turn the crockpot on, you can cook on the high setting for two to four hours (depending on the meat) but don't leave it unattended.

Note that all ingredients are given in per-meal amounts for one 50-pound dog, and all amounts can be adjusted for multiple meals, dogs, and/or varying body weights.

Bison Stew

1 cup ground bison (ground beef may be substituted)
¼ cup chopped broccoli or celery (generally, feed ¼ cup veggies per meal)

Add water and cook in a crockpot on low setting 6 to 8 hours.

When cooled, add serving of bison and vegetables to food bowl along with another protein source: either a cooked egg, a raw organic egg with chopped shell, or ¼ to ½ cup plain yogurt, lassi or kefir. Since bison is low in fat, add 1-2 teaspoons of hempseed oil to provide both omega-3 and omega-6 fatty acids. Make sure to add the crockpot broth to the meal!

Chicken Deluxe

> 1-1½ cups chicken breast or thighs (Remove skin if dog has a weight issue. Debone before feeding and discard bones so that dogs can't get them out of the garbage.)
> 1-2 tablespoons chicken liver
> ¼ - ½ cup chopped carrots or string beans
> ¼ cup sliced sweet potato with skin (optional)
>
> Add water and cook in a crockpot on low setting.
>
> When cooled, put serving of chicken, vegetable, sweet potato, and broth from the crockpot in food bowl, along with 1 teaspoon of flaxseed oil or chia seeds.

Surf and Turf

> 1 cup chopped beef roast
> ¼ cup green peas
> ⅛ cup sliced apples (optional)
>
> Add water and cook in a crockpot on low setting.
>
> In a food processor blend 1 can of sardines (with skin and bone in water or olive oil).

Mix beef and vegetable/fruit with sardines. Add the broth from the crockpot.

Turkey Time

> 1 cup ground turkey
> ¼ cup cauliflower, chopped
> 1 tablespoon fresh or dried basil or oregano

Add water and cook in a crockpot on low setting.

When cooled, add serving of turkey and vegetable to food bowl along with ½ cup yogurt, lassi, kefir, cottage cheese, or 1 egg (cooked or organic, raw with crushed shell). Add 1 teaspoon flaxseed oil or 1 teaspoon chia seeds. You can add a teaspoon of blueberries if you like. Add broth from the crockpot.

Beef and Chicken

> 1½ cups ground beef and chicken breast mix
> ¼ cup vegetable of your choice.

Add water and cook in a crockpot on low setting.

As an alternative to adding vegetable to the beef and chicken, you can add 1 tablespoon of oregano or basil, fresh or dried. When the crockpot cooking is done, you can add ¼ cup canned organic squash to your dog's meal. Squash doesn't do well in a crockpot for hours, but can be added later from a can or after steaming.

You will need to balance the fats; camelina oil's balance of omega-3 and omega-6 fatty acids (plus high vitamin E) make it perfect for this combination of proteins. Feed 1-2 teaspoons for a 50-pound dog.

Venison or Elk

(When you have the opportunity to feed these wild ruminants, they provide excellent food for dogs.)

1.5 cups ground venison or elk

Add water, turn crockpot on low.

In the last hour of cooking, add ¼ cup chopped kale. When cooled, add serving of venison or elk with the kale to food bowl and add 1-2 teaspoons of hempseed oil. Optionally, you can add 1 tablespoon organic pumpkin meal. Add broth from the crockpot.

Mixing raw and cooked

- You can mix cooked bison with raw bison (1 cup cooked with ¼ - ½ cup raw).

- You can mix cooked chicken with raw turkey or chicken necks.

- You can mix cooked salmon with either raw ground bison, or several tablespoons of raw organ meat (beef heart or beef liver).

- You can add commercially prepared raw foods to your cooked meal (see Appendix C's "Seeking the Balance" entry for recommendations).

- Remember, don't be afraid of real food!

How about grains?

I personally avoid grains with my dogs unless I need to bulk up the GI tract with rice to address diarrhea or stomach upset. Chicken and rice is an old standby for most vets, but I don't favor grains as a daily food for my dogs.

Some holistic vets do like oatmeal—not daily, but just as an added, alternative source of fiber. Cooked, whole oats, oat groats, or organic oat bran may be used, with the reminder that dogs need more protein and fat than they do fiber and carbohydrates.

Appendix B: More Tips on Feeding Raw

There are some wonderful informational resources available for making and feeding raw food meals for your dog. My favorites are:

- *The BARF Diet* by Dr. Ian Billinghurst
- *Unlocking the Canine Ancestral Diet* by Steve Brown
- *Raw and Natural Nutrition for Dogs* by Lew Olson, PhD
- *Dogs Naturally Magazine's How To Make Raw Dog Food: A Primer*

If you're going to make raw food meals for your dog, you will want to consult these resources!

There are also a number of YouTube videos on raw feeding. Here are some of my favorites that were available on the site as of October, 2017:

- "The Perfect Seven-Day Raw Feeding Plan for Dogs": *https://www.youtube.com/watch?v=Brfqbzj4Uv4*

- "Raw Dog Food Tutorial": *https://www.youtube.com/watch?v=2u8L7Xav1-8*

- "Raw Meat Diet for Dogs and Cats": *https://www.youtube.com/watch?v=G3wLTlqnMMg*

- "Raw Food Diet for Dogs and Cats": https://www.youtube.com/watch?v=ijP_CVZUa5g

Bones and chews

"Raw meaty bones" (RMBs) are important to the raw diet because they provide critical minerals like calcium and phosphorus, and nutrients such as glucosamine and cartilage. Raw bones are completely digestible. *Never feed cooked bones, EVER.* Cooked bones are indigestible because cooking changes the structure of the bone. Cooking also makes bones brittle; fragments can get stuck in the esophagus, in the dog's lower jaw, or lodge in the stomach or intestines.

The best raw meaty bones are chicken wings, chicken necks, chicken backs and turkey necks. Beef and lamb ribs are tougher compared to chicken bones but are good for variety. You want the meat on the bones because it helps the dog slow down and chew. Some raw food feeders also feed turkey necks. A wonderful source of glucosamine and cartilage are dehydrated chicken feet, or duck feet, which are especially beneficial to the arthritic dog.

I do give my dogs beef knuckle bones or marrowbones twice a week. These bones are extremely tough, and for an aggressive chewer could break or crack a tooth. My dogs are more interested in getting at the marrow and bits of meat on the bone, and really aren't all that interested in chewing it. When the dogs are finished, I take the bones and make bone broth.

Note that there are some dog breeds known as *brachycephalic* ("shortened head") whose teeth and jaw conformations may not be compatible with raw meaty bones. These include the boxer, bulldog, pug, and shih tzu among others.

Chews are great for teeth cleaning. My dogs love beef trachea, and beef or bison tendon chews. I generally order chews like these online from Springtime, Inc. and raw dog food companies also may offer trachea and tendon chews

Worried about feeding raw bones whole?

If you're hesitant to feed raw bones whole, and want to make your own raw food, then you will need to invest in a meat grinder. Here are two that are often recommended:

- The Weston Pro Series No. 22 Commercial Meat Grinder (pricier)

- The STX Magnum 1800W Meat Grinder (less expensive, but not strong enough to do turkey necks)

Alternatives to making your own raw dog food

Sometimes it's a lot easier to buy commercially prepared raw dog food. It's more expensive than making your own, so you have to consider convenience versus cost. My favorite brands are: *Stella & Chewy's, Tucker's, Oma's Pride, Steve's Real Food, My Pet Carnivore, Miami Raw, ReelRaw,* and *Darwin's Natural Pet Products*. What I especially like about these companies is that ground bone and organ meat is part of the food.

How much to raw to feed?

The basic rule of thumb is to feed, per day, 1 to 2 percent of the dog's body weight. So if your dog weighs 50 pounds, you would feed approximately ½ to 1 pound of food per day. Raw food weighs more than kibble since it has moisture, bones, and organ meats.

Adding a multivitamin/mineral

Whether you decide to go with home-made raw, commercial raw, or a combination of the two, you do want to add a whole-food multivitamin/mineral. Raw food is not fortified as kibble is (with vitamins from less-than-desirable sources like petroleum and coal tar). A whole-food multi-nutrient formula will ensure your dog is getting all the necessary vitamins, minerals, and antioxidants he or she needs.

Listen to your intuition

One of the most important aspects of feeding and caring for dogs is listening to your intuition. No one knows your dog better than you do. Sometimes, however, it is not our intuition speaking—it is our fears. I've found that I need to step away, take a walk, sit quietly somewhere, and sort out my intuitive feelings from my fear feelings. I ask myself: *what am I afraid of?* Whatever comes to mind, I may write down, or just let the thoughts come through, without judgment. Letting the fears out makes room for our intuition to speak.

There have been many times I did not listen to my intuition and deeply regretted tuning out. One example I will never forget was with a rescue dog named Possum. He was a Lab puppy that had been found with his sister tied to a tree. The shelter volunteers named him Possum because he was shy. I adopted him and when he was just over a year old my intuition told me that something wasn't right with him. My mind searched for evidence: his stool, appetite, energy, attitude, and could see nothing out of normal. Perhaps two or three days later he had a funny look in his eyes, but everything else about him was normal. My intuition was now screaming at me, but my brain said, "There's nothing wrong...look at how happily he's playing." Less than a week later, he had projectile black diarrhea. I rushed him to the vet where he was diagnosed with liver disease and, despite surgery, he didn't make it.

Sample home-made raw recipes

The number one favorite home-made raw food meal with the Aussie Tribe is sardines. Canned sardines aren't strictly "raw" but are steamed and sometimes lightly smoked. You can find true raw, fresh-caught sardines at some specialty stores. This recipe is based on feeding one meal to five dogs of approximately 50 pounds each.

Sardines Supreme

In a food processor, add:
4 cans of sardines with bones (in water or olive oil). Each can is 4.2 ounces, and most of the dogs get a whole can, but because two of my Aussies have to watch their waistlines, I divide 1 can between the two of them (about 2 ounces each).
¼ cup chopped kale for each dog, or 2 tablespoons per dog of organic canned or cooked squash or organic canned pumpkin
2 tablespoons of blueberries per dog
Blend well.

Once I have divided the servings into the food bowls, I will add another protein: either a raw egg with chopped shell or cottage cheese (around ½ cup) plus some raw bison meat (¼ to ½ cup per dog). You will notice your dog eats this meal in nanoseconds.

Ruminant Beef

This recipe, adapted from *Unlocking the Canine Ancestral Diet* by Steve Brown, will feed a 25-pound adult dog for one week or a 50-pound dog for four days.

In a food processor, add:
4 pounds 90-93% lean ground beef
¾ pound ground beef heart, preferably grass-fed
¼ pound beef liver, preferably grass-fed
1 pound squash, lightly cooked or finely ground raw
  (The original recipe substitutes spinach here,

although I personally don't feed it. Spinach may not be tolerated well by some dogs, particularly those with kidney problems, and it is high in purines that can lead to excessive accumulation of uric acid.)

½ pound broccoli stalks or other vegetable, lightly cooked or finely ground raw

1 can of sardines in water

1½ ounces of human-grade bone meal (*I use ground egg shells*)

4 teaspoons hempseed oil

2 teaspoons iodized salt (*I use sea salt*)

Blend well and refrigerate.

Appendix C: Product Recommendations

The literature and products listed in this section are arranged by chapter for easy reference.

Chow Time: What to Feed Dogs

An excellent collection of raw food recipes can be found in the book *Chow Hounds* by Ernie Ward, DVM.

When adding fats to your dog's diet, BioStar recommends the Nordic Pet product line from manufacturer Nordic Naturals, because of the high quality of their oil processing.

Dog Food Allergies

When feeding raw to address allergies, our favorites include:

- Tucker's Raw Frozen & Treats
- Stella and Chewy's Frozen Raw Dinners
- Oma's Pride Raw Food
- Primal Pet Foods' Pronto Formulas
- Raw Feeding Miami
- My Pet Carnivore

- ReelRaw

Visit www.dogfoodadvisor.com/best-dog-foods/raw-dog-food/ for many more commercially available raw food suggestions.

Feeding the Overweight Dog

Among other diet-friendly options, I choose Wholistic Pet Organics Sea Kelp, as it provides important minerals and nutrients and helps speed up metabolism by supporting the thyroid.

As for low-fat treats, BioStar's Dog Star Liver Treats are an excellent choice, along with Stewart freeze-dried Pro-Treat products—made from 100% beef liver and nothing else.

Feeding for Healthy Skin and Coat

For the sample rotation feed plan, we recommend Stella & Chewy's chicken/duck/turkey patties, and the beef/pumpkin patties available from Tucker's Raw Frozen. There are also excellent ground whole prey (including organs and bones) that you can order online from ReelRaw, Steve's Real Food, My Pet Carnivore, and Raw Feeding Miami.

For getting clean and conditioned, the Pet Shampoo & Conditioner from Warhorse Solutions is my top pick for coat and skin. It contains glycerin, coconut oil, raw sunflower oil, castor oil, avocado oil, almond oil, dead sea salt and several other essential oils: tea tree, lemon, citronella, lemongrass, wood of rose, and lavender. This shampoo moisturizes, cleans, and nourishes skin and hair...*and* the dogs don't smell like they just stepped out of a French red light district.

Feeding for the Kidneys

For kidney support, we recommend BioStar's Optimum K9 multivitamin/mineral, along with BioStar's Terra Biota K9: a full-spectrum, high-potency probiotic/prebiotic supplement for dogs with 1.5 billion CFUs per serving.

For omega-3 and omega-6 fatty acid supplementation, Nordic Naturals Fish Oil for dogs is a great choice. (Due to concern over levels of mercury and other toxins in fish oils, the company recommends contacting them for certificates of analysis that guarantee purity.)

Feeding for the Liver

The source of a nutrient is important, especially for dogs with liver or other health issues. Vitamins that are petroleum-sourced or made from coal tar just put more stress on the GI tract.

Among food-sourced vitamins, BioStar's Optimum K9 multivitamin/mineral is an excellent option for providing vitamins E and A, along with the vitamin C and B complex support that's crucial for liver health.

Feeding for the Pancreas

Low-fat plain yogurt is helpful toward eliminating fat from the diet and keeping a beneficial bacterial balance in the GI tract. On days when you don't feed yogurt, give a multi-strain, active probiotic with at least one billion CFUs per serving, such as BioStar's Terra Biota K9.

Feeding the Diabetic Dog

Camelina oil is an excellent source of fatty acids and vitamin E for dogs with diabetes, and we recommend BioStar's Gold Star K9. It's unrefined, never heat-processed, and provides an ideal 2:1:1 ratio of the omega-3, 6, and 9 fatty acids, along with vitamin E alpha, beta, and gamma tocopherols. Vitamin E is an important antioxidant that assists with normal inflammatory response for dogs.

Feeding Dogs with Cancer

Stewart Pro-Treat freeze-dried beef liver treats are perfect snacks for dogs with cancer. As for supplements, the following are all good, whole-food dietary support options:

- BioStar's Optimum K9 contains *spirulina* for macro- and micro-minerals plus phytonutrients and antioxidants. In addition, Optimum K9 provides nutritional yeast for B vitamins and additional protein.

- The medicinal mushroom complex (reishi, shiitake, cordycepts, maitake) included with BioStar's Terra Biota K9 formulation is important for immune support.

- BioStar's Colostrum-38 K9 is a high-potency bovine colostrum for immune report and cellular repair.

- Fish oil from Nordic Naturals is good for the essential fatty acids, with purity backed up by certificates of analysis available on request. If you're still concerned about contaminants in fish oil, use a high-quality camelina oil (such as BioStar's Gold Star version), which not only supplies high levels of omega-3, but the antioxidant vitamin E as well.

For making CBD oil (or other plant butters or extracts) try the Magical Butter Botanical Extractor Machine, available through Amazon and other outlets.

Feeding Puppies

As mentioned, www.dogfoodadvisor.com is an excellent resource for feeding puppies of all breed sizes. So is the online publication *Dogs Naturally* Magazine.

If you choose to go raw with your large or giant-breed puppy, you should look into a book by Dr. Ian Billinghurst called "Grow Your Pups with Bones", as well as a *Dogs Naturally* article found at www.dogsnaturallymagazine.com/starting-puppy-on-raw-diet/. In general, this magazine is a great source of raw feeding and nutritional information that I highly recommend.

Among supplements for puppies, I use BioStar's Optimum K9 cubes for a multivitamin option because they're 100% whole food and bite-size, so you can give them as treats. BioStar's Terra Biota is my choice for multi-strain probiotic, and Nordic Naturals is my preferred supplier of fish oils.

Seeking the Balance

There are a number of books with recipes for raw food diets that can help make feeding raw both fun and less mysterious. Two of my favorites are: *Dinner PAWsible* by Cathy Alinovi, DVM, and *The BARF Diet* by Dr. Ian Billinghurst.

In terms of commercial raw food, today's options are better than ever. For those of us who are time-pressed and are only able to make a raw meal once or twice per week at best, there are some great convenient pre-prepared frozen raw formulas available.

These are the brands I've personally used and often feed in rotation:

- Steve's Raw Food
- Tucker's Raw Frozen
- Stella and Chewy's freeze-dried Meal Mixer SuperBlends
- Primal Pet Foods
- Darwin's Natural Pet Products
- Raw Feeding Miami
- My Pet Carnivore
- ReelRaw

Dog Food Advisor is an excellent online resource for its rating system, applied to many companies' products. Not all raw dog foods have been rated by Dog Food Advisor, but Stella & Chewy's, Primal, Tucker's and Steve's have been.

If you choose to make your own raw meals, there are some excellent videos and articles on how to feed raw available at dogsnaturallymagazine.com.

Warming, Cooling, and Neutral Foods

Ayurvedic principles are the foundation of BioStar's Topper formulations: whole-food blends of dehydrated and freeze-dried food designed to be added on top of your dog's meals.

Buckaroo's Stew: Warming formula can be added to kibble, raw food, canned food, and home cooked food, and can be hydrated by adding water or broth. This warming formula is perfect for chilly winter days or for older dogs throughout the year.

Buckaroo's Stew: Cooling formula is perfect for hot summer days or for dogs that are very active throughout the year. This blend supplies the Ayurvedic balancing and cooling foods that provide variety to your dog's diet, support the various populations of the gut microbiota, and satisfy the innate canine curiosity over new tastes and smells.

Bovine Colostrum for Canines

Bovine colostrum is measured by its IgG content, which can range from 10 to 40% (with the highest content generally used as a milk replacement for calves and foals). BioStar's Colostrum-38 K9 is a 38%, freeze-dried colostrum produced in Canada from grass-fed cows that are r-BGH-free and antibiotic-free. Due to its high IgG content and high bioactivity, serving sizes are small—a little goes a long way.

Supplements

There is a powdered version of turmeric with ground black pepper and powdered coconut oil on the market called Turmericle from Stance Equine. It also includes the antioxidant *resveratrol*. If you don't want to make golden paste, this is an easy and very palatable alternative.

In the realm of calming supplements, BioStar's Thera Calm K9 is a unique complex for promoting calmness for dogs that become upset or anxious during times of stress. Made into handy cubes, it's a blend of milk casein, herbs, brewer's yeast, organic pumpkin, organic coconut oil, organic flax seeds, and desiccated liver that makes a nourishing and tasty supplement. Can be used every day or as needed.

The Puppy Cometh

At home, Wookie the Puppy gets supplemented with BioStar's Optimum K9 powder multivitamin/ mineral, and rewarded with Dog Star Liver Treats. The easy-to-handle bully stick rings she loves to chew are sold by Barkworthies.

Acknowledgements

This book would not be possible without the support of a very special group of people: *Rick, Lynn, Leslie, Jamie, Elva, Lindsey, Emily, JP, Judy,* and *Jolene.* Thank you for everything you do for BioStar, and on behalf of all the dogs and horses we make products for.

Thank you to *Bernie McMahon* for your wise counsel, insights, and great dog stories.

A special thanks to breeder, judge, and trainer *Lori Fausett* and your Soundtrack Australian shepherds. Thank you for your guidance, mentorship, and the privilege of owning five of your wonderful dogs.

Thank you to my partner-in-crime, Peter, who makes my life wonderful in so many ways.

Thank you to *Dave*, my editor, whose emails I initially dread, but then am grateful for. Couldn't do this without you.

Thank you to *Karen* at All Things Pawssible in Charlottesville for your amazing insight and understanding of all things canine.

And lastly, to the Springdale Pack—Kemosabe, Thunderbear, Mr. Schmoo, Crockett, and Wookie—as well as all the dogs I've shared a lifetime with. Thank you for being such patient teachers.

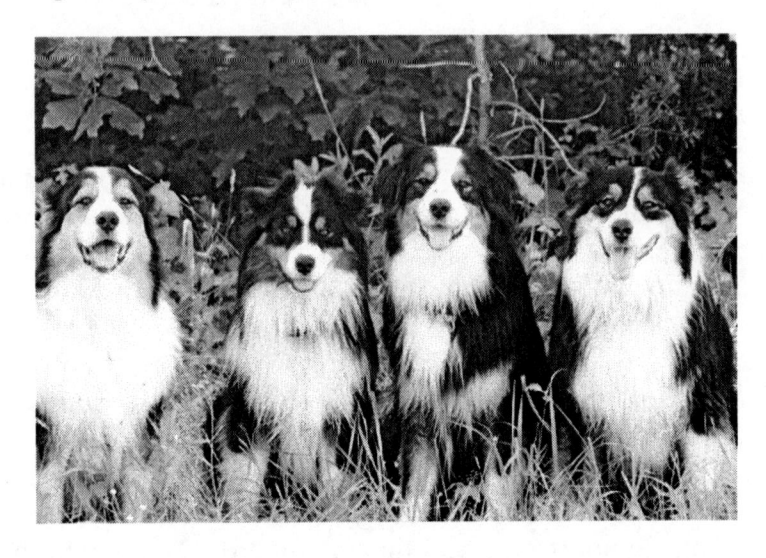

Bibliography

Alinovi, Cathy. *Dinner PAWsible*. Skyhorse Publishing, 2015.

Bhattacharyya, Sumit et al. "Increased expression of colonic wnt9A through sp1-mediated transcriptional effects involving arylsulfatase B, chondroitin 4-sulfate, and galectin-3." *The Journal of Biological Chemistry*, American Society for Biochemistry and Molecular Biology, 20 June 2014, www.ncbi.nlm.nih.gov/pmc/articles/PMC4067192/.

Billinghurst, Ian. *The BARF Diet*. Dogwise Publishing, 2001.

Brønden, L B. "Data from the Danish veterinary cancer registry on the occurrence and distribution of neoplasms in dogs in Denmark." The Veterinary Record, U.S. National Library of Medicine, 8 May 2010, www.ncbi.nlm.nih.gov/pubmed/20453236.

Brown, Steve. *Unlocking the Canine Ancestral Diet*. Dogwise Publishing, 2009.

Byrne, Jane. "EFSA draws a blank on safety of ethoxyquin use in feed." Feednavigator.com, William Reed Business Media, Ltd. 19 Nov. 2015, www.feednavigator.com/Article/2015/11/19/EFSA

-draws-a-blank-on-safety-of-ethoxyquin-use-in-feed.

Dyck, Amy. "24 Bad Dog Food Ingredients to Avoid." Homes Alive Pets Blog, Homes Alive, Ltd., 28 Sept. 2015, www.homesalive.ca/blog/bad-dog-food-ingredients-to-avoid/.

Féher, J, and G Lengyel. "Silymarin in the prevention and treatment of liver diseases and primary liver cancer." Current Pharmaceutical Biotechnology, U.S. National Library of Medicine, Jan. 2012, www.ncbi.nlm.nih.gov/pubmed/21466434.

Fleck, A, et al. "Anti-arthritic efficacy and safety of Crominex® 3 (trivalent chromium, *Phyllanthus emblica* extract, and shilajit) in moderately arthritic dogs." *Journal of Veterinary Science & Animal Husbandry*, Annex Publishers, 16 Sept. 2014, www.annexpublishers.com/blog/anti-arthritic-efficacy-and-safety-of-crominex-3-trivalent-chromium-phyllanthus-emblica-extract-and-shilajit-in-moderately-arthritic-dogs-3/.

Hadhazy, Adam. "Think twice: How the gut's 'second brain' influences mood and well-being." *Scientific American*, Nature America, Inc., 12 Feb. 2010, www.scientificamerican.com/article/gut-second-brain/.

International Agency for Research on Cancer. "Glyphosate." *IARC Monographs on the Evaluation of Carcinogenic Risks to Humans.* World Health Organization, 2016, http://monographs.iarc.fr/ENG/Monographs/vol112/mono112-10.pdf

Leighton, Robert. *The New Book of the Dog.* Cassell & Company, Ltd., 1906.

Lenox, CE, Bauer, JE et al. "Potential adverse effects of omega-3 fatty acids in dogs and cats." *Journal of Veterinary Internal Medicine.* 2013; 27(2): 217-226.

Olson, Lew. *Raw and Natural Nutrition for Dogs.* North Atlantic Books, 2010.

Scott, Dana. "Healing golden turmeric paste recipe for your dog." *Dogs Naturally Magazine.* DNM, Inc., 3 May 2017, www.dogsnaturallymagazine.com/healing-with-turmeric-golden-paste-for-dogs/.

Scott, Dana. "The disturbing cause of dental disease in dogs." *Dogs Naturally Magazine*, 11 May 2017, www.dogsnaturallymagazine.com/the-disturbing-cuase-of-dental-disease-in-dogs/.

Scott, Dana. "Starting Your Puppy On A Raw Diet." *Dogs Naturally Magazine*, DNM, Inc., 20 June 2017, www.dogsnaturallymagazine.com/starting-puppy-on-raw-diet/.

Steinberg, Steven (Coordinator). Veterinary Cancer Registry. Veterinary Specialty Services, LLC, 2017. www.vetcancerregistry.com/.

Syme, Bruce. "Digesting Bones, Gastric Acidity, Salmonella in Dogs and Cats." Vet's All Natural, 27 Sept. 2017, www.vetsallnatural.com.au/digesting-bones-gastric-acidity-salmonella/.

ter Veld, Marcel G.R. "Estrogenic potency of food-packaging-associated plasticizers and antioxidants as detected in ERα and ERβ reporter gene cell lines." *Journal of Agricultural and Food Chemistry*, ACS Publications, 20 May 2006, pubs.acs.org/doi/abs/10.1021/jf052864f.

Thixton, Susan. "Who makes what in pet food." Truth About Pet Food, 21 Mar. 2013, truthaboutpetfood.com/who-makes-what-in-pet-food/.

Thurston, Mary Elizabeth. *The Lost History of the Canine Race*, 1st ed. Andrews McMeel, 1996.

Tudor, Ken. "More study results from the nutrition symposium." PetMD, Pet 360 Media Network, www.petmd.com/blogs/thedailyvet/ktudor/2013/june/more-nutrition-studies-from-research-symposium-30509.

U.S. Food & Drug Administration. "Code of Federal Regulations Title 21." Accessdata.fda.gov, 1 Apr. 2017, www.accessdata.fda.gov/scripts/cdrh/cfdocs/cfcfr/cfrsearch.cfm?fr=101.22.

Vaughn, DM et al. "Evaluation of effects of dietary n-6 to n-3 fatty acid ratios on leukotriene B synthesis in dog skin and neutrophils." *Veterinary Dermatology*. 1994; 5(4): 163-173.

Walsh, John Henry. *The Dog in Health and Disease*, 4th ed. Ballantyne Press, 1887.

About the Author

Tigger Montague has spent her entire life with dogs, either purchased from breeders, rescued, or adopted from shelters. Living with multiple dogs taught her pack behavior, and she began to see her dogs as members of a tribe: a Chief, the Elders, the Storyteller, the Hunters, and the Hearth-Seekers. After 30 years in the human and equine nutrition business, she embarked on her own journey for foods that could nourish and support members of the canine tribe. Her company, BioStarUS, has pioneered whole, raw food supplements for dogs and horses.

Index

2,4-D, 175
AAFCO, 91, 92, 104
Acana, 122
acetaminophen, 164
agility, xi, 102, 112
Ainsworth Pet Nutrition, 122
Akita, 174
algae, 110, 113, 208
Alinovi, 292, 299
allergies, 89, 97, 127, 146, 287
almonds, 213
amino acids, 97, 101, 109, 110, 111, 121, 128, 139, 217
ammonia, 157, 158
amylase, 167
ancestral diet, 197, 208
animal byproduct, 90, 92
antacids, 164
antibiotics, 201, 202, 230
anti-inflammatory, 140, 148, 216, 220
antioxidant, 94, 95, 104, 113, 148, 161, 180, 181, 217, 220, 221, 282, 290, 291, 295, 302
apple cider vinegar, 150, 254, 269

apples, 7, 80, 113, 131, 153, 158, 159, 212, 213, 274
Armour, 119
arsenic, 116
arthritis, 136, 211, 213, 219
Ascorbates, 111
ashwaganda, 147, 221
astaxanthin, 113, 131
ATP, 208
Australian cattle dog, 68
Australian shepherd, xi, xii, 24, 39, 42, 43, 44, 51, 61, 82, 251, 262
autolyzed yeast, 98
AuxiGro, 97
Ayurvedic medicine, 211, 215, 232
bacteria, 145, 167, 199, 204, 216, 217, 233
bananas, 212
BARF Diet, 279, 292, 299
Barkworthies, 295
barley, 102, 103, 105, 107, 108, 119, 166, 167, 170, 212
basset hound, 174
beagle, 169, 174
Bear Dog, vii, xiii, 59, 60, 184
beef meal, 114
beet pulp, 105

307

benzene, 175
Bernese mountain dog, 174
Berwind Corp., 122
beta carotene, 171
BHA, 90, 93, 94, 95
Bhattacharyya, Sumit, 299
BHT, 90, 93, 94, 95
bichon frise, 174
Bifidobacteria, 217
Big Heart Pet Brands, 124
Billinghurst, Ian, 299
bioavailability, 110, 113
BioStar, xii, 183, 219, 287, 288, 289, 290, 291, 292, 294, 295, 297
bison, 53, 114, 115, 117, 129, 141, 144, 166, 167, 176, 177, 178, 179, 189, 213, 229, 230, 273, 276, 281, 284
bladder, 151, 173, 244, 257
bloating, 127
blood meal, 93
blood urea nitrogen, 151
bloodhound, 174
blue heeler, 68
blueberries, 113, 115, 129, 131, 153, 154, 158, 159, 213, 275, 284
boar, 129, 139, 141
bone broth, 53, 89, 136, 150, 178, 179, 219, 271, 280
bone meal, 92, 153, 285

bones, 53, 89, 91, 93, 115, 117, 118, 124, 129, 134, 149, 150, 153, 176, 177, 179, 188, 189, 191, 193, 194, 198, 204, 208, 251, 269, 270, 271, 272, 274, 280, 281, 282, 284, 288, 302
border collie, 65
boswellia, 147, 220
boxer, 68, 174, 281
brachycephaly, 281
brain, 30, 51, 98, 140, 199, 283, 300
brain-gut connection, 111, 199
bran, 92, 106, 212, 277
branched-chain amino acids, 102
broccoli, 97, 131, 158, 159, 166, 167, 171, 176, 178, 179, 212, 273, 285
Brønden, LB, 174, 299
Brown, Steve, 279, 284, 299
Brussels sprouts, 176
Buckaroo, xii, 51, 54, 62, 63, 80, 195, 233, 240, 245, 249, 257, 258, 265, 269, 294
Buckaroo's Stew, 294
buffalo, 89, 122, 129, 134, 139, 166, 170
bulldog, 65, 281
bullmastiff, 174
Bully Dog, 75, 76, 77, 78

Byrne, Jane, 94, 299
cabbage, 119, 153, 158, 166, 167, 170, 176
cadmium, 116
cairn terrier, 169
calcium, 109, 110, 129, 153, 188, 208, 217, 280
calcium caseinate, 99
California, 89, 123, 175
calming supplements, 221, 295
calories, 108, 114, 129, 134
camelina, 116, 125, 129, 136, 142, 143, 171, 180, 190, 192, 213, 276, 290, 291
Campylobacter, 204
Canada, 31, 104, 145, 294
Canadian timber wolf, 12
cancer, 94, 145, 157, 163, 173, 174, 175, 176, 177, 182, 183, 184, 209, 291, 299, 300, 301, 302
cannabidiol, 182
cannabis, 14, 182, 183, 184
capric acid, 142
caprylic acid, 142
carbohydrates, 101, 106, 107, 108, 112, 114, 128, 158, 163, 167, 169, 170, 176, 191, 204, 207, 208, 277
Cargill Animal Nutrition, 91
carrageenan, 99, 155
Carrie, 76, 77, 78

cartilage, 216, 280
cats, xii, xiii, 1, 17, 39, 55, 66, 67, 90, 104, 175, 235, 237, 239, 240, 241, 252, 253, 265, 267, 272, 301
cauliflower, 153, 154, 159, 176, 212, 275
Cavalier King Charles spaniel, 174
CeeCee, 23, 24, 25, 27, 28, 31, 33, 36, 37
celery, 97, 115, 150, 158, 159, 270, 273
cellulose, 106
certificate of analysis, 116
chelates, 110, 111
Chesapeake Bay retriever, 174
chews, 192, 280, 281
chia, 129, 142, 143, 213, 274, 275
chicken, 21, 45, 54, 55, 58, 61, 62, 63, 66, 80, 81, 89, 90, 92, 97, 98, 102, 104, 110, 117, 125, 127, 128, 129, 134, 139, 142, 143, 150, 153, 154, 155, 158, 159, 166, 170, 176, 177, 178, 179, 189, 193, 201, 202, 211, 212, 229, 258, 269, 270, 271, 274, 275, 276, 280, 288
chicken byproduct, 93

chickens, xii, 1, 53, 54, 58, 61, 62, 89, 101, 104
Chihuahua, 174
Chile, 207
Chow Chow, 24, 169
Christmas Stew, 269, 272
chromium, 219, 300
citric acid, 99
CJ Foods, 122
cleaners, 146, 175
Clostridium, 201, 204
coal tar, 109, 113, 160, 208, 282, 290
coat, 24, 47, 66, 68, 139, 140, 142, 143, 147, 190, 205, 254, 262, 289
cocamide, 144
cocker spaniel, 164, 174
coconut, 104, 106, 116, 125, 129, 134, 136, 142, 144, 147, 153, 154, 177, 179, 181, 182, 190, 193, 213, 220, 221, 289, 295
cod, 159
collagen, 129, 149, 188
collard greens, 166, 167, 176, 179
colostrum, 130, 131, 147, 180, 215, 216, 217, 218, 220, 291, 294
Colostrum-38 K9, 291, 294
combination diet, 111, 114
commands, 194

cooling foods, 211, 212, 213, 294
copper, 157, 217
CoQ10, 229
corgi, 66, 67, 68
corn, 77, 90, 92, 99, 102, 103, 104, 107, 109, 111, 127, 136
cortisol, 221, 262
cottage cheese, 125, 134, 136, 158, 159, 165, 166, 170, 171, 176, 177, 179, 189, 213, 275, 284
couscous, 158, 159
coyotes, xii, 83, 207
creatine, 151
Crockett, xii, 51, 61, 63, 81, 83, 187, 195, 201, 218, 225, 227, 232, 240, 243, 244, 249, 252, 257, 264, 297
crockpot, 89, 129, 135, 149, 150, 178, 179, 191, 269, 270, 273, 274, 275, 276
Crominex 3+, 219
cucumbers, 97, 153, 158, 159
Cujo, 36, 37
curcumin, 181
Cushing's disease, 164
cysteine, 139
cystine, 139
cytokines, 216, 217
dachshund, 169
dairy, 96, 109, 127, 139, 158
Dalmation, 65

Darwin's Natural Pet Products, 282, 293
deer, xii, 15, 45, 46, 47, 106, 255
dehydration, 151, 155
dermatitis, 144, 145, 146
detoxification, 149
DHA, 116, 140, 142
diabetes, 78, 105, 108, 163, 164, 169, 290
Diamond Pet Foods, 122
diarrhea, 127, 151, 163, 201, 212, 214, 233, 262, 266, 277, 283
diazolidinyl urea, 144
dioxins, 105
dirt, 86, 145, 239, 255
disodium guanylate, 99
disodium inosinate, 99
diuretics, 164
Doberman pinscher, 169, 174
Dog Food Advisor website, 114, 189, 288, 292, 293
Dog Star Liver Treats, 288, 295
Dogs Naturally magazine, 279, 292, 301
drugs, 90, 118, 230
dry food, 155
ducks, 59, 60
Dyck, Amy, 99, 300
dyes, 90, 127
dysplasia, 134, 188

E. coli, 204
ear infection, 127
eggs, 34, 54, 66, 81, 109, 115, 124, 131, 144, 153, 154, 159, 165, 166, 167, 170, 171, 177, 178, 179, 189, 212, 229, 258, 259, 273, 275, 284, 285
elk, 129, 139, 141, 276
emulsifiers, 96, 127
endocrine system, 145, 221
English, Doug, 181
enteric nervous system, 199, 200
enzymes, 109, 121, 128, 147, 163, 167, 191, 198, 230
EPA, 116, 140, 142
ethanol, 106
ethoxyquin, 90, 93, 94, 299
ethylene oxide, 145
excitotoxin, 98
extrusion, 120, 121
eyes, 140
fascia, 137
fats, 90, 93, 95, 104, 116, 121, 128, 134, 136, 139, 140, 141, 143, 145, 157, 163, 192, 207, 276, 287
fatty acids, 103, 105, 116, 121, 139, 140, 141, 142, 143, 171, 180, 219, 274, 276, 290, 291, 301
feather meal, 127
Féher, J, 161, 300

fiber, 101, 105, 106, 108, 111, 112, 116, 134, 135, 158, 207, 208, 233, 262, 270, 277
fibrogenesis, 161
Finnish spitz, 169
Firmicutes, 199
fish, 53, 93, 94, 101, 102, 103, 105, 109, 110, 113, 114, 116, 127, 129, 139, 142, 158, 171, 180, 192, 211, 212, 289, 291, 292
fish meal, 93, 114
flavor enhancers, 95, 127
flavorings, 90, 96, 155
flax, 104, 116, 125, 134, 143, 159, 192, 213, 295
flea collars, 90, 102
flea-and-tick dip, 175
Fleck, A, 219, 300
food intolerance, 127, 129, 191
food processor, 115, 136, 274, 284
formaldehyde, 144
foxes, 15, 61, 62, 255
free-choice feeding, 112
free-range, 66, 115, 159, 229
frozen, 111, 125, 134, 150, 182, 189, 193, 293
gas, 127
gastritis, 163
gelatin, 99, 149, 188
genetics, 146, 173, 188, 209

German shepherd, 12, 33, 59, 174
GI tract, 89, 128, 129, 136, 143, 146, 147, 149, 160, 165, 167, 173, 181, 183, 190, 191, 192, 199, 202, 203, 204, 205, 211, 212, 214, 229, 231, 233, 258, 262, 263, 266, 277, 290
GLA, 183
glucosamine, 149, 150, 219, 280
glucose, 163, 169, 219
glutamate, 97, 99
glutamic acid, 99
glycemic index, 108
glycine, 149
glycosaminoglycan, 149
glyphosate, 175
GMOs, 104, 106, 107, 111, 173
goat's milk, 193, 208, 213
Gold Star K9, 290
golden paste, 181, 220, 221, 295
golden retriever, 169, 174
goose, 129
gooseberries, 219
grain-free, 90, 107, 108, 147
grease, 95
Great Dane, 157, 174
Great Pyrenees, 174
green beans, 106, 125, 135, 150, 193, 211

green peppers, 97
greyhound, 174
growth factors, 130, 215, 217, 218, 220
gut, 136, 147, 149, 198, 199, 204, 300
gut bacteria, 199, 217, 294
gut microbiome, 146
Hadhazy, Adam, 200, 300
hair, 105, 139, 144, 191, 289
Hawkeye, vii
heart, 92, 166, 167, 170, 178, 179, 276, 284
heat stress, 212
heavy metals, 105, 116
hempseed, 104, 113, 116, 124, 129, 141, 144, 273, 276, 285
herbivores, 152
herding, xi, 7, 8, 22, 39, 65, 66, 68, 102, 112, 255, 265
herring, 103
hexane, 104, 109
Hill's Pet Nutrition, 91
hives, 127, 145
holidays, 60, 265, 266, 269
holy basil, 147, 262
home-cooked food, 2, 101, 111, 113, 124, 125, 130, 134, 135, 136, 155, 158, 176, 177, 185, 187, 189, 191, 197, 198, 204, 205, 208, 219
homeostasis, 151, 218, 221

hooves, 127
hormones, 127, 230
horse meat, 120
hot spots, 127, 146
Hungarian Puli, 169
hunting dogs, 102, 112
hyaluronic acid, 149
hydrolyzed protein, 97, 98, 99
hydrolyzed yeast, 97, 98
hypercalcemia, 153
imidazolidinyl urea, 144
immune system, 128, 130, 131, 146, 173, 215, 216, 217, 249
immunoglobulins, 130, 216, 217
inflammation, 113, 128, 136, 146, 147, 163, 164, 181, 183, 212, 213, 214
insulin, 105, 163, 169, 215
International Agency for Research on Cancer, 175, 301
intestines, 92, 93, 191, 280
intuition, 214, 282, 283
Irish wolfhound, 174
isopropyl alcohol, 106, 144
itching, 127
Japan, 94, 145
Jar Jar Binks, vii, 41
JoJo, 33
kale, 53, 109, 115, 134, 148, 150, 154, 166, 171, 176,

179, 208, 212, 270, 276, 284
kaolin clay, 262
Keeshond, 169
kefir, 53, 89, 124, 129, 147, 153, 154, 178, 189, 191, 192, 201, 208, 219, 233, 270, 273, 275
kelp, 131, 134, 135, 171, 219, 288
Kemosabe, xi, 1, 2, 52, 83, 133, 135, 136, 194, 201, 223, 232, 269, 297
kibble, 90, 95, 111, 112, 114, 117, 118, 119, 120, 121, 124, 128, 129, 135, 143, 147, 149, 155, 173, 187, 188, 189, 190, 191, 192, 198, 200, 204, 205, 207, 208, 209, 257, 282, 294
kidneys, 94, 151, 152, 155, 163, 165, 166, 167, 173, 178, 179, 209, 285, 289
kiwi fruit, 212
Kizzie, vii, 66, 67, 68
Kojak, vii
krill, 116
Labrador retriever, 59, 157, 169, 266
lactating, 102
Lactobacillus, 217
lactoferrin, 217
lamb, 7, 110, 114, 127, 141, 165, 176, 178, 179, 280
lassi, 89, 124, 178, 179, 208, 219, 231, 232, 233, 262, 270, 273, 275
laureth sulfate, 145
lauric acid, 130, 142
lauryl sulfate, 145
lead, 116
leaky gut syndrome, 149
legumes, 105, 109, 139
Leia, 24, 25, 26, 27, 28, 29, 31, 32, 33, 34, 35, 36, 37
Leighton, Robert, 119, 301
Lenox, CE, 301
lentils, 158
leptin, 98
lettuce, 53, 212
Lhasa apso, 65
lipase, 167
liver, 94, 101, 130, 136, 149, 157, 158, 159, 160, 161, 163, 165, 166, 167, 170, 173, 178, 179, 180, 181, 193, 209, 220, 231, 258, 274, 276, 283, 284, 288, 289, 290, 291, 295, 300
livestock feed, 91
macronutrients, 130, 154
Magical Butter Botanical Extractor Machine, 291
magnesium, 188, 217
Malamute, 12, 13, 169
maltodextrin, 99
mangoes, 212
Mars Petcare, 123

massage, 137
mastiff, 174
MCI, 145
meat byproduct, 90, 121, 208
meat fibrine, 117
meat grinder, 281
Medicated Dog Bread, 117
Mei Mei, vii, xiii
mercury, 105, 116, 171, 289
methionine, 102, 139
Mexico, 207
micronutrients, 130, 154
microorganisms, 146, 147, 192, 233
milk, 89, 117, 118, 153, 154, 176, 179, 189, 191, 192, 213, 231, 294, 295
milk thistle, 160
Milk-Bones, 124, 192
millet, 153
minerals, 101, 109, 110, 111, 113, 129, 135, 142, 171, 180, 207, 208, 217, 269, 280, 282, 288, 291
miniature pinscher, 169, 174
miso, 107
molasses, 35, 112
Monsanto, 94, 175
MSG, 97, 98, 99
multivitamin, 113, 130, 154, 160, 190, 192, 208, 219, 258, 282, 289, 290, 292, 295

mushrooms, medicinal complex, 180, 291
My Pet Carnivore, 281, 287, 288, 293
myristic acid, 142
National Research Council, 91, 107
natural flavors, 96, 97, 98, 99
nausea, 60, 127
necks, 129, 176, 193, 271, 276, 280, 281
Nestlé Purina, 91
neurotoxin, 104, 109
neutering, 133
neutral foods, 211, 213, 214, 294
Newfoundland, 174
Nikki, vii
Nordic Naturals, 287, 289, 291, 292
North Carolina, 25, 78, 184
NSAIDs, 181, 184
Nutro Products, 91
nuts, 105, 107, 139, 212
oatmeal, 119, 144, 153, 158, 159, 166, 167, 277
oats, 102, 103, 105, 107, 108, 118, 170, 213, 277
obesity, 108, 169, 199
oils, 90, 96, 104, 105, 109, 113, 115, 116, 124, 125, 129, 130, 134, 136, 141, 142, 143, 144, 145, 147, 153, 154, 158, 159, 171,

177, 179, 180, 181, 182, 183, 184, 190, 192, 193, 212, 213, 220, 221, 254, 273, 274, 275, 276, 284, 285, 287, 289, 290, 291, 295
Old English sheepdog, 169
older dogs, 218, 294
Olson, Lew, 279, 301
Oma's Pride Raw Food, 281, 287
omnivores, 101, 152
organ meats, 89, 153, 166, 179, 192, 282
organophosphates, 164
Orijen, 122
orthopedic disease, 188
osteochondrosis (OCD), 188
overweight dogs, 98, 108, 112, 133, 135, 142, 164, 175, 194, 202, 226, 288
palmitic acid, 142
Panacur, 202
pancreas, 163, 164, 165, 166, 167, 169, 170, 290
pancreatitis, 157, 163, 164, 165, 167
papayas, 213
papillon, 174
parabens, 145
parasite, 146
pasta, 212
peaches, 212
peanuts, 212

pears, 212
peas, 105, 129, 144, 176, 211, 270, 274
pectin, 99, 106
Pekingese, 174
pepper, black, 181, 182, 220, 221, 295
performance dogs, 112, 113, 218
pesticides, 94, 106, 107, 157, 173, 175, 203
Peter, xii, xiii, 40, 48, 49, 50, 51, 56, 57, 61, 62, 81, 82, 83, 133, 225, 226, 263, 297
petroleum, 109, 145, 155, 160, 175, 208, 244, 282, 290
phosphorus, 110, 129, 151, 152, 153, 155, 188, 208, 217, 280
picky-eater syndrome, 89, 129, 191
piperine, 181
polyethylene glycol, 145
polysorbate, 145
pomace, 106
Pomeranian, 174, 250
poodle, 20, 65, 164, 169, 174
poop, 198, 205, 230, 263
pork, 103, 153, 165, 176, 178, 179, 229
Possum, 283
possums, xii, 101, 255
potassium, 151, 217

potatoes, 97, 105, 108, 119, 127, 176, 212, 270
poultry, 95, 96, 102, 103, 104, 127, 139, 142, 158, 165, 166, 190
prebiotics, 289
prednisone, 164
preservatives, 90, 93, 94, 96, 127, 128, 145, 173, 208
Primal Pet Foods, 287, 293
probiotics, 147, 154, 167, 192, 217, 219, 231, 232, 233, 262, 289, 290, 292
Proctor & Gamble, 123
proline-rich polypeptides, 130, 216
propyl gallate, 90, 94
propylene glycol, 90, 95, 145
protease, 99, 167
protein, 91, 92, 96, 97, 98, 101, 102, 103, 105, 108, 110, 113, 114, 116, 127, 128, 129, 139, 144, 145, 147, 151, 152, 157, 158, 163, 165, 167, 169, 170, 180, 190, 204, 208, 216, 217, 229, 273, 277, 284, 291
proteinates, 110, 111, 113
psyllium, 106
pug, 281
pumpkin, 89, 106, 115, 124, 129, 131, 134, 143, 153, 154, 158, 166, 167, 189, 193, 194, 198, 201, 202, 213, 233, 262, 270, 276, 284, 288, 295
puppies, 1, 68, 102, 146, 187, 188, 189, 190, 191, 192, 193, 194, 195, 257, 259, 292
puppy classes, 194, 195
Quaker Oats, 119
quaternium-15, 144
quinoa, 107, 153, 211
rabbit, 89, 139, 190, 212
Ralston Purina, 119, 120
rash, 127
Ravenwolf, vii, xiii, 12, 77
raw food, 111, 115, 128, 134, 143, 147, 176, 188, 189, 191, 198, 199, 200, 204, 246, 258, 271, 279, 280, 281, 283, 287, 288, 292, 293, 294
rawhide, 192, 193
ReelRaw, 281, 288, 293
rendering, 95, 102, 104, 136, 158, 208
resveratrol, 221, 295
riboflavin, 217
ribs, 161, 176, 190, 280
rice, 89, 102, 106, 107, 119, 127, 153, 154, 158, 159, 166, 167, 170, 201, 202, 211, 277
ringworm, 35

Rocky Raccoon, vii, xiii, 7, 68, 69, 72, 73, 253
rosemary, 131
Rottweiler, 36, 174
Roundup, 175
Royal Canin, 123, 133, 200, 202, 203
ruminants, 141, 276
Rutrow, vii, 79, 253
rye, 105, 107
Saint Bernard, 174
salmon, 89, 103, 129, 141, 142, 143, 159, 171, 177, 190, 192, 212, 229, 276
Salmonella, 201, 204, 302
Samoyed, 169
sardines, 89, 110, 115, 125, 129, 136, 141, 142, 143, 144, 153, 176, 177, 179, 189, 198, 211, 274, 275, 283, 284, 285
Scandinavia, 174
schipperke, 169
schnauzer, 164, 169, 174
Schylur, vii
Science Diet, 200
Scott, Dana, 301
selenium, 217
Sergeant Major, The, 10, 20, 21, 22
serotonin, 200
sesame, 212
shampoo, 144, 146, 255, 289
shea butter, 144

Shetland sheepdog, 174
shiba inu, 65
shih tzu, 174, 281
shilajit, 219, 300
Siberian Husky, 24, 69
Sierra, vii, 12
silymarin, 161
skin, 105, 106, 119, 127, 134, 139, 140, 143, 144, 145, 146, 147, 158, 159, 166, 170, 179, 215, 216, 225, 249, 274, 289, 303
skunks, 45, 253, 254, 255, 256
Skye Dog, vii, 7, 8, 9, 10
sled dogs, 102, 112
socialization, 75, 195, 259
sodium, 151, 217
sodium caseinate, 98
soil, 53, 107, 145
sorbitol, 95
soy, 90, 97, 98, 103, 104, 107, 110, 127, 136
SPCA, 1, 8, 39, 48, 59, 67
Spike, vii, 65
spinach, 110, 166, 167, 170, 176, 284
Spirit Dog, vii, xiii, 39, 40, 41, 42, 44, 45, 46, 47, 48, 49, 50, 51, 52, 57, 73, 79, 244, 253, 254, 262, 263
spirulina, 113, 131, 148, 171, 180, 291
sporting dogs, 102

Spratt's, 117, 118
springer spaniel, 169
squash, 154, 166, 170, 171, 176, 178, 179, 189, 193, 194, 213, 275, 284
Star Wars, 23, 250
starch, 99, 121, 165, 176
Steinberg, Steven, 302
Stella and Chewy's, 287, 293
Stewart Pet, 288, 291
stomach, 105, 163, 204, 205, 261, 277, 280
strawberries, 97, 131, 212
stress, 30, 42, 113, 128, 146, 147, 149, 157, 160, 165, 173, 192, 221, 251, 259, 261, 262, 263, 290, 295
sugar, 95, 105, 106, 163, 232
summertime, 213
superoxide dismutase, 217
supplements, xii, 98, 109, 110, 113, 131, 133, 142, 147, 180, 219, 221, 291, 292
sweet potatoes, 89, 129, 131, 153, 154, 166, 176, 213, 270, 271
Sweetie, 12, 15, 16, 20, 21, 22, 62
Swift, 119
Syme, Bruce, 205, 302
tapioca, 153, 154
teeth, 114, 129, 191, 202, 281
tempeh, 107

ter Veld, Marcel, 94, 302
Terra Biota K9, 289, 290, 291
tetracycline, 164
tetrahydrocannabinol (THC), 183
Thera Calm K9, 295
thiamine, 217
Thixton, Susan, 122, 302
Thunderbear, xii, 51, 54, 62, 63, 81, 83, 85, 86, 195, 196, 226, 240, 245, 249, 252, 257, 258, 259, 262, 263, 264, 266, 297
Thurston, Mary, 118, 302
thymus, 130, 147, 216
thyroid, 133, 135, 144, 219, 288
Toby, vii, 66, 67
tocopherols, 290
tofu, 107
toluene, 175
tomatoes, 60, 77, 78, 97, 106, 253, 254
toxins, 145, 146, 149, 151, 157, 173, 193, 220, 262, 289
training, 13, 194, 195, 259
transferrin, 217
triclosan, 146
tripe, 153, 154
trout, 129
TruthAboutPetFood.com, 122

Tucker's Raw Frozen, 287, 288, 293
Tudor, Ken, 152, 302
Tufts Registry, 174
turkey, xii, 59, 60, 89, 103, 110, 129, 139, 142, 143, 150, 159, 167, 176, 177, 193, 211, 212, 265, 275, 276, 280, 281, 288
turmeric, 147, 181, 182, 220, 221, 295, 301
Turmericle, 221, 295
USFDA, 96, 303
variety, importance of feeding, 125, 129, 134, 139, 143, 199, 229, 280, 294
Vaughn, DM, 303
venison, 15, 89, 129, 134, 139, 141, 144, 178, 179, 212, 269, 276
veterinarian, 98, 107, 127, 128, 133, 151, 157, 161, 163, 169, 181, 184, 200, 201, 203
vitamins, 101, 109, 113, 121, 155, 160, 171, 180, 207, 208, 217, 258, 276, 282, 289, 290, 291
vomiting, 127, 151, 163
Walsh, John Henry, 118, 303
Warhorse Solutions, 289
warming foods, 211, 213, 214

watermelon, 97, 212
weight loss, 82, 136
WellPet, 122
West Highland white terrier, 169
wheat, 90, 92, 106, 107, 109, 118, 127, 211
wheat grass, 212
Wholistic Pet Organics, 288
Winter Equestrian Festival, 243
wintertime, 207
wolves, xi, 101, 105, 207, 230
Wookie, vii, 7, 24, 25, 26, 27, 28, 29, 30, 31, 32, 33, 34, 35, 36, 37, 38, 189, 251, 257, 258, 259, 260, 295, 297
working dogs, xii, 102
World Health Organization, 175, 301
worms, 202
xylene, 175
yeast, 96, 97, 98, 127, 180, 233, 291, 295
yeast extracts, 98
Yoda, 250, 251, 252
yogurt, 89, 124, 129, 136, 147, 154, 158, 159, 165, 166, 167, 170, 171, 177, 179, 192, 219, 231, 273, 275, 290
Yorkshire terrier, 164
YouTube, 279

zinc, 217

zucchini, 78, 134, 158, 166, 170, 176, 178, 179, 213

CPSIA information can be obtained
at www.ICGtesting.com
Printed in the USA
FFOW05n0441021217